MISSIONS OF THE USAF
COMBAT CONTROL TEAMS:

To employ by air-land-sea tactics into forward, non-permissive enviroments to establish assault zones with an Air Traffic Control capability.

To establish recovery zones for surface to air recovery of personnel or equipment.

To provide ground-based fire control for AC-130 gunship operations.

To provide command and control radio capabilities in the forward area.

As needed, to clear obstructions and hazards with demolitions.

MISSIONS OF THE USAF
PARARESCUE TEAMS:

To deploy by air-land-sea tactics into forward non-permissive environments and provide trauma medical care.

To participate in search and rescue (SAR) and combat search and rescue (CSAR).

As needed, to act as aircrew gunners and/or scanners on both fixed and rotary wing aircraft.

ACKNOWLEDGMENTS

We would like to thank the following individuals and organizations for their time, effort, and support:

Air Force Public Affairs
Colonel Ronald T. Strand
Director
Pentagon, Washington, DC

Mr. Doug Thar
Senior Account Executive
Pentagon, Washington, DC

Lackland Air Force Base, TX
Mrs. Irene Witt
Media Relations Director
Office of Public Affairs

Brig. Gen. Barry Barksdale
Commander
37th Training Wing

Col. Kenneth Freeman
Commander
37th Training Group C

Lt. Col. David Corwin
Commander
342nd Training Squadron

Major John Hennessey
Commander
342nd Training Squadron Combat Training Flight

Master Sgt. Rodney Alne
Superintendent
342nd Training Squadron Combat Flight Training

Master Sgt. Craig Showers
Commandant
342nd Training Squadron PJ/CCT School

Our editorial consultants: Nathalie Zimmerman and Susan Ruszala
Our design and production team:
Dede Cummings and Gary Szczecina
And to the many others who contributed to the success
of this mission: thank you!

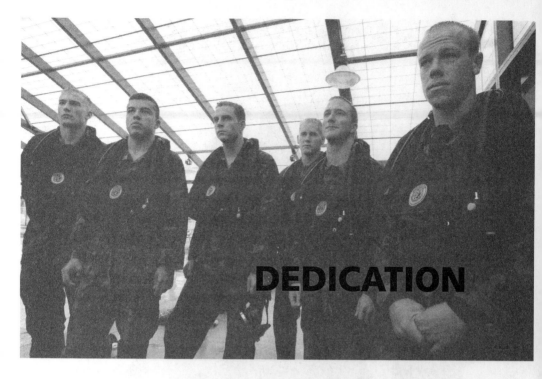

DEDICATION

To the PJs and CCTs—past, present, and to come. Your self-sacrificing dedication is acknowledged and commended. Your heroism serves as a shining example for all Americans.

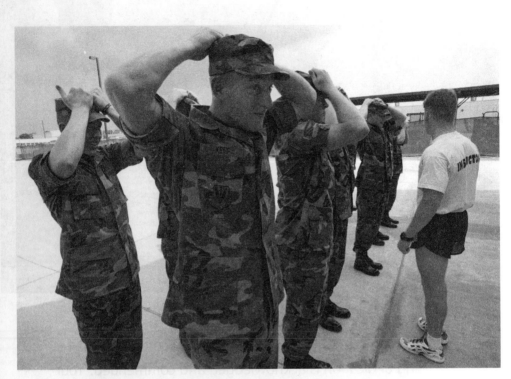

Fixing hats during uniform inspection, Lackland AFB, Texas.

CONTENTS

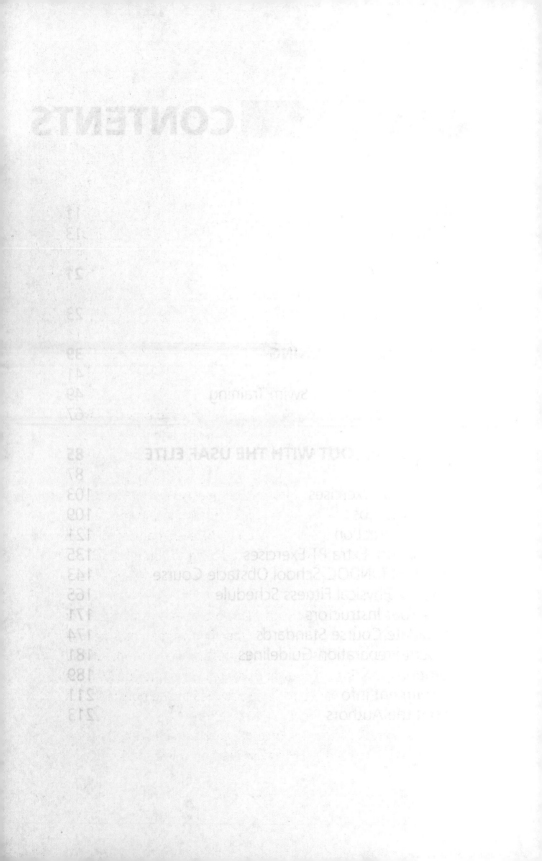

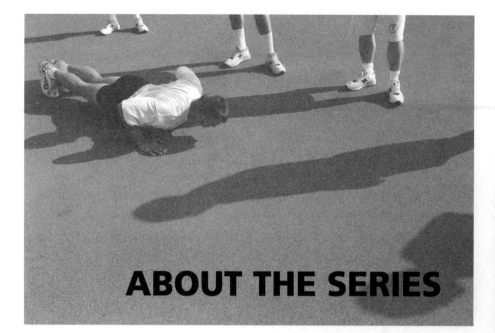

ABOUT THE SERIES

The Five Star Official Fitness Guides are designed to provide a fresh new perspective on the subject of personal health and fitness by documenting the physical training regimens of the United States Armed Forces.

To bring you this exciting information, we have shouldered our gear in the hot midday sun, on cold frosty mornings, in the dark of night. No workouts and training schedules were reorganized to meet our needs. Nor did we ask. We wanted to bring to you what's REAL. We like to think of these books as "fitness documentaries" —because that's what they are!

We have talked extensively with many individuals responsible for the physical fitness and welfare of the men and women of America's Armed Forces. We have discovered the most powerful workout and physical training routines in the world. We bring them to you with the hope that you will be inspired to value your health and pursue fitness activities throughout your life.

Wherever possible, primary source material is utilized. Documentation, interviews, briefs—all were assembled and culled for details and insights.

Important note: These books are not designed to be follow-to-the-letter workouts. That was never our intention. These books are a collection of information on the subject of fitness and physical training in the US military, full of techniques, routines, hints, suggestions, and tips you can learn from. Your workout should be individualized. We highly recommend you review your fitness plan with a certified trainer, coach, or other individual who possesses the proper knowledge to advise you in such a manner. And of course, consult your physician before commencing any new fitness program or before you intensify your current regimen.

**Good luck and may lifelong fitness
be your goal!**

Andrew Flach
Peter Field Peck

INTRODUCTION

Welcome to the Five Star Fitness look at the elite Air Force training of the Pararescuemen and Combat Controllers, the fifth book in our continuing series on military fitness. In these pages you'll find details on one of the most vigorous and demanding training regimens known to man. Developed with the assistance of the US Air Force, this book delivers the most comprehensive and thorough presentation of the physical training programs unique to the Pararescue and Combat Control units.

The Pararescue units, or PJs, of the United States Air Force are responsible for providing emergency and life-saving services to airmen, soldiers, and civilians in both peacetime and combat environments. When a plane goes down—as it did recently in Yugoslavia—it is the Air Force's Pararescue team who are there to find and save American pilots. Pararescuemen truly live up to their motto, "That Others May Live."

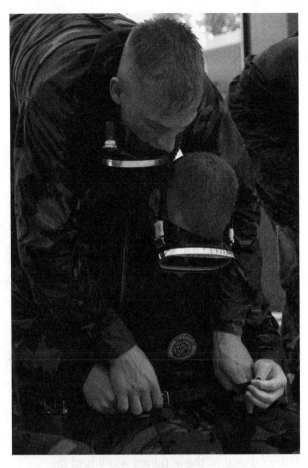

Combat Control Technicians, or CCTs, have a motto too: "First There." This motto derives from the fact that the CCTs are able to infiltrate into a designated area by almost any imaginable means. Once they have reached the target area, they provide ground force commanders with vital communications, command and control links between aircraft commanders and rear headquarters commanders. They have the ability to perform an essential function unmatched by any other airborne unit—air traffic control service, day and night, even under the most difficult conditions.

Both pararescue and combat control team members receive extensive training in a multitude of areas: parachute operations, waterborne infiltrations, mountain operations, helicopter operations, overland movement, and arctic operations. Their training—which you will find detailed extensively in this book—includes "drownproofing," running 50 miles per week, weight training, calisthenics, and more. Taking on the challenge of becoming a PJ or CCT is not for the weak of heart!

ELIGIBILITY REQUIREMENTS

To be eligible to become a PJ or CCT, you must:

- Be a US citizen.

- Be a volunteer.

- Be a male (based on current Department of Defense policies).

- Have a general score of at least 43 on the Armed Services Vocational Aptitude Battery test.

- Be able to pass a Class III flight physical (done during basic military training).

- Have vision of no worse than 20/100, correctable to 20/20.

- Have normal color vision.

- Be able to obtain a secret security clearance (done during basic military training).

- Meet specific physical fitness standards.

- Be a high school graduate or have a General Education Development certificate.

- You must attain a score of at least 100 points on the Physical Ability and Stamina Test (PAST), to be completed during basic training.

- You must be a proficient swimmer.

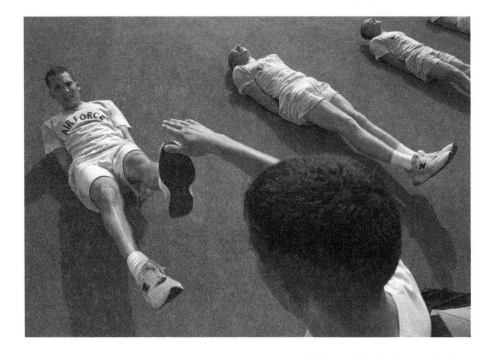

If you're interested in becoming a PJ or CCT, this is the book for you. In these pages you'll find actual training schedules used in the Pararescue/ Combat Control Candidate Course. These workouts are designed to allow you to achieve the minimum standard requirements to pass the Candidate Course. In addition to preparing you physically with training schedules and details on proper exercise techniques (including swimming), we've tried to prepare you mentally for the rigorous training you'll face. We've presented you with an in-depth look at the water confidence and swim training methods used by instructors to help build students' confidence in themselves. And you'll take a step-by-step journey through the famous Obstacle Course that every candidate must conquer. These are only a few of the many areas we've covered in this book.

If you're not interested in joining the PJs or CCTs, this book will provide you with an excellent training program—convenient, simple,

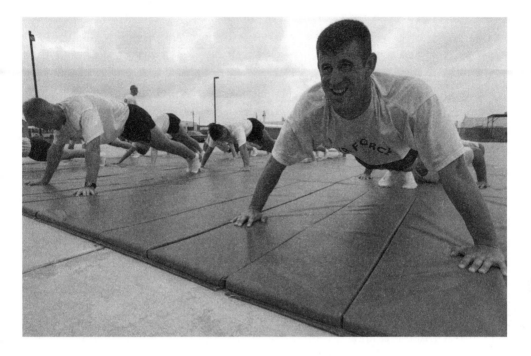

THE MISSION

"It's pitch black outside. Our aircraft slows to jump speed and the ramp quickly lowers. Everyone is tense as we near the release point. Fifteen seconds from "green light" the jumpmaster gives us "thumbs up." We make last second adjustments to our equipment packs, altimeters, and goggles. The green light flashes on. The jumpmaster points outside the aircraft and shouts "GO" over the interteam radio. Out we go into the cold darkness at 18,000 feet. The adrenalin is pumping, but we're all well trained and ready for action. Our mission—survey an airfield without being detected by enemy forces."

–from US Air Force Combat
Controller literature

and effective. With a combination of calisthenics, upper and lower body exercises, abdominal exercises, running, and weight training, you will be well on your way to achieving maximum physical fitness. The techniques and methods used by the US Air Force are proven and reliable—there are no gimmicks or fancy equipment used here. Only a commitment to fitness and a desire to achieve are necessary.

This book is structured in six parts. Parts I and II provide an introduction to the PJs and CCTs. You'll learn how these elite Air Force teams came to be, and the important role they've played in crises throughout the world. We've documented the training requirements to become a PJ or CCT, from the Pararescue/Combat Control Candidate Course to the different pipelines you can follow once you complete basic training. Part III is an inside look at the fitness training candidates must master—run training, water confidence and swim training, and the weight circuit. Take a look at this chapter if you're interested in what the candidates really endure. Or, check out Part V, the Obstacle Course. These 21 obstacles are definitely challenging!

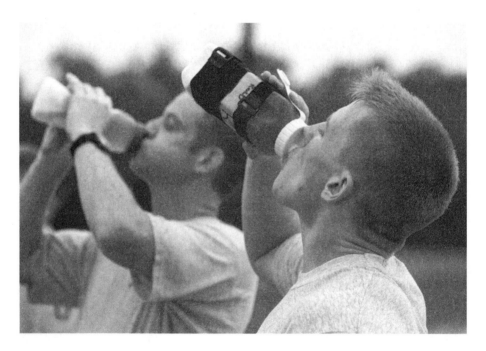

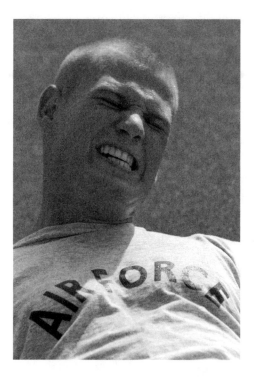

Part IV is a closer look at the stretches, upper and lower body exercises, pull-ups and dips, and ab workouts PJs and CCTs perform. It's here that you'll learn to "do them right." You'll be glad you did, cause you'll definitely be cranking out quite a few situps, pushups and pull-ups! We've finished up in Part VI with some authentic workout schedules used by real PJs and CCTs in training. Rigorous and draining, these workouts will prepare you for the Candidate Course—and get you in the best shape of your life!

The workouts included in this book are tough, without a doubt. But the rewards and benefits you'll gain from looking back and saying to yourself, "Hey, I did that!" are immeasurable. Every time you complete a particularly challenging day of exercises or an extra-long run you'll be increasing your confidence and pride in yourself. The PJs and CCTs have to be prepared to be confident and strong in the face of unthinkable danger, and their training isn't only intended to build muscles and increase endurance. The future PJs and CCTs enrolled in the Candidate Course learn teamwork, trust, and leadership skills—skills almost as necessary in the field as strength and endurance.

Our journey with this book introduced us to many great people. Above all, we came away from the experience with the belief that the members of the US Air Force Elite, the Pararescuemen and Combat Controller Technicians, deserve great respect and admiration. They do a job many would avoid, and as quiet professionals, most people will never know the jobs they've done or the great risks they've encountered.

We hope that this book will leave you with the same admiration we've experienced, along with a strong plan for achieving maximum physical fitness. Good luck! And to those members of US Air Force Elite teams who courageously serve our nation: We thank you! God Bless.

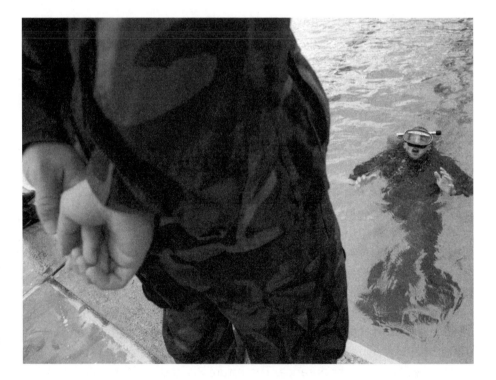

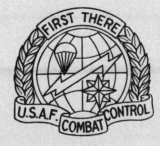

PART I

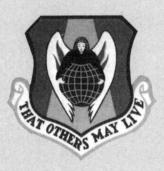

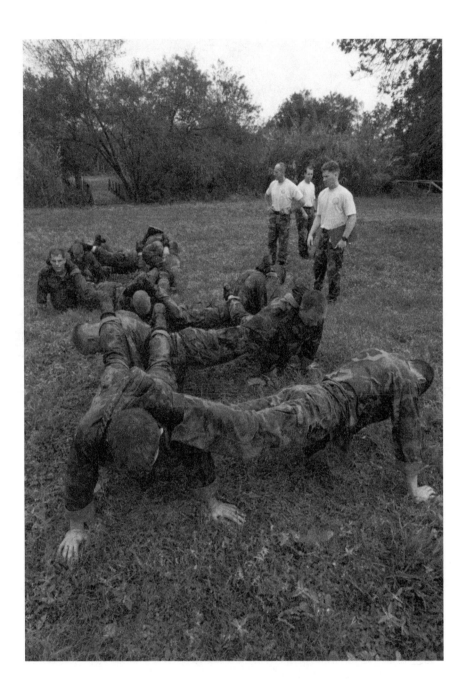

WHO ARE THE PARARESCUEMEN AND COMBAT CONTROL?

Who are the Pararescuemen and Combat Control?

Imagine the only way to save a life was to jump from a plane and parachute into uncharted, possibly hostile, jungle terrain with 150 pounds of gear.

Not only do you have to be able to save a life but you have to clear the way for incoming aircraft to locate you and land. For the average person, this sounds absolutely terrifying and virtually impossible, but for the Pararescue and Combat Control units of the United States Air Force, this is what they train for. Nothing stands in the way of the Pararescue and Combat Control teams when it comes to saving lives—it's their primary mission.

The United States Air Force Pararescue unit (PJs) are an elite group of highly trained professionals who perform life-saving missions in some of the world's most remote locations. The primary responsibility

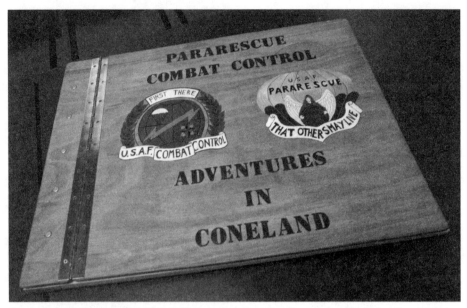

Each day during the PJ/CCT INDOC course, the class is required to submit a cartoon reflecting the previous days events. PJ/CCT trainees are referred to as "coneheads" and the instructors are known as "sharks." The best of these cartoons are preserved in a series of albums known as "The Adventures in Coneland".

of the PJs is to provide emergency medical treatment to airmen, soldiers, and civilians in both peacetime and combat environments. They are highly trained emergency trauma specialists, which requires them to maintain at least Emergency Medical Technician (EMT) Intermediate or a higher qualification throughout their careers. Pararescuemen are trained in air, land, and sea tactics, which they utilize to take them into a designated territory and deliver medical care to the injured. To reach casualties, Pararescuemen may take part in search and rescue (SAR), combat search and rescue (CSAR), or any other necessary operations.

There are no commissioned officers among the PJs ranks. All are enlisted or non-commissioned officers (NCOs).

Combat Controller Technicians (CCTs) work hand-in-hand with Pararescue units to establish the critical communications link between ground and aircraft commanders. CCTs establish assault zones in specific areas that are either drop zones (for parachute landings), landing zones (for fixed wing or helicopter operations), or extraction zones (for low altitude re-supply). As needed upon reaching their destination, CCTs might clear an airfield, position navigation aids, and set up air traffic control for inbound aircraft. Or they may also establish ground to air recovery zones—for personnel or equipment—and ground-based fire control for gun operations. The CCTs are highly skilled air traffic controllers, the capabilities of which require exhaustive technical training recognized by the Federal Aviation Administration (FAA).

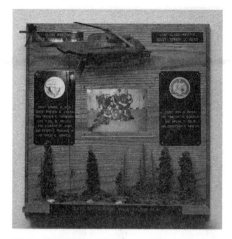

Every PJ/CCT INDOC graduating class presents the school with a plaque. The plaques can often be complex, as this model shown above, or can be humorous. One class presented a surf board as their plaque. Another class presented a life size fiberglass shark (see page 173).

A BRIEF HISTORY OF THE PARARESCUE UNITS

The origin of the modern day PJs can be linked to a remote crash site near the China-Burma border in August of 1943. Twenty-one men were in desparate need of rescue after having bailed out of their disabled C-46. Surrounded by rugged terrain and dense jungle, the only way of getting the help and medical attention they needed was by paradrop. This event stressed the need for a team of highly trained rescue specialists and thus, the PJs came to be.

Pararescuemen retrieved Gemini 8 astronauts David Scott and Neil Armstrong from a successful splashdown in the Pacific.

Throughout numerous events since their inception, the PJs have demonstrated valiant displays of heroism during times of both conflict and peace.

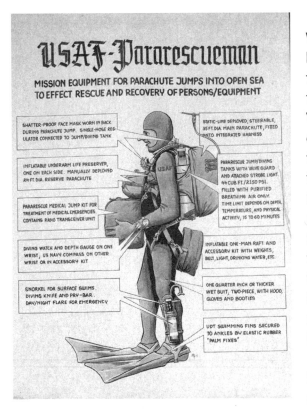

USAF-Pararescueman

MISSION EQUIPMENT FOR PARACHUTE JUMPS INTO OPEN SEA TO EFFECT RESCUE AND RECOVERY OF PERSONS/EQUIPMENT

SHATTER-PROOF FACE MASK WORN IN BACK DURING PARACHUTE JUMP. SINGLE-HOSE REGULATOR CONNECTED TO JUMP/DIVING TANK

INFLATABLE UNDERARM LIFE PRESERVER, ONE ON EACH SIDE. MANUALLY DEPLOYED 24 FT. DIA. RESERVE PARACHUTE

PARARESCUE MEDICAL JUMP KIT FOR TREATMENT OF MEDICAL EMERGENCIES. CONTAINS RADIO TRANSCEIVER UNIT

DIVING WATCH AND DEPTH GAUGE ON ONE WRIST, US NAVY COMPASS ON OTHER WRIST OR IN ACCESSORY KIT

SNORKEL FOR SURFACE SWIMS, DIVING KNIFE AND PRV-BAR. DAY/NIGHT FLARE FOR EMERGENCY

STATIC-LINE DEPLOYED, STEERABLE, 35 FT. DIA. MAIN PARACHUTE, FITTED ONTO INTEGRATED HARNESS

PARARESCUE JUMP/DIVING TANKS WITH VALVE GUARD AND ATTACHED STROBE LIGHT. 44 CUB. FT./2150 PSI. FILLED WITH PURIFIED BREATHING AIR ONLY. TIME LIMIT DEPENDS ON DEPTH, TEMPERATURE, AND PHYSICAL ACTIVITY, IS 10 TO 60 MINUTES

INFLATABLE ONE-MAN RAFT AND ACCESSORY KIT WITH WEIGHTS, BELT, LIGHT, DRINKING WATER, ETC.

ONE QUARTER INCH OR THICKER WET SUIT, TWO-PIECE, WITH HOOD, GLOVES AND BOOTIES

UDT SWIMMING FINS SECURED TO ANKLES BY ELASTIC RUBBER "PALM FIXES"

During the Vietnam War, the PJs risked their lives to aid wounded infantrymen and pilots in the hostile territory of the Vietnamese jungle. In early 1966, the PJs were formally recognized by the Air Force Chief of Staff and received approval to wear the maroon beret, symbolizing the blood they sacrifice in their devotion to saving lives and living up to their motto, "That Others May Live."

Other historical events in which PJs played a significant role included 1989 Operation Just Cause in Panama and the action for the liberation of Kuwait, Operation Desert Storm. In addition to rescue missions in Desert Storm, PJs also provided extensive support for airlift operations providing relief to Kurdish refugees fleeing into northern Iraq.

PJs were also involved in the struggle to capture Somali leader Mohammed Fhara Aidid, during which they rescued injured aircrewmen from the midst of fierce fighting.

The life-saving deeds of the PJs have taken them to the sea, bringing them to the aid of downed pilots, merchant seamen, and civilians alike. Today, PJs continue to provide support to the National Aeronautics and Space Administration's (NASA) Space Shuttle program.

In 1989, Pararescuemen were personally recognized by then President George Bush for their efforts in recovering and treating victims of the devastating San Francisco earthquake.

A BRIEF HISTORY OF COMBAT CONTROL

The need for Combat Controllers first became apparent during airborne campaigns of World War II, when major parachuting assaults fell short of expectations due to lost aircraft and adverse weather. The result was the creation of a small parachute force which would precede the main assault force to the objective location and provide critical visual guidance and weather information to inbound aircraft.

These Army Pathfinders, as they were called, were employed in September of 1943 during the airborne reinforcement of allied troops in Italy, and further demonstrated their effectiveness during the Normandy invasion, and the September 1944 airborne operation code-named Market Garden, in which units of the 101st Airbone and 82nd Rangers dropped behind enemy lines into Holland to secure key strategic bridgeheads.

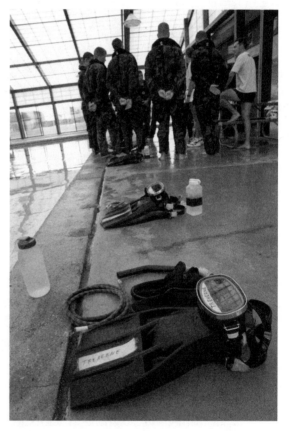

In September 1947, the US Air Force was officially recognized as a separate branch of the United States Armed Forces. Prior to this time, military aviation was controlled by the Army Air Corps. Due to this fundamental re-alignment of the US military, the Pathfinder teams, later called Combat Control, sustained a series of organizational changes.

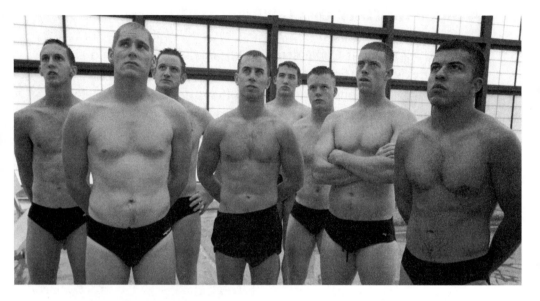

CCT units were formally activated in January of 1953 to provide navigational aid and air traffic control for airlift forces. The restructuring of the CCT units underwent their last change in 1991 when they were placed under the control of host wing commanders.

Since their initial activation into the United States Air Force, CCTs have played an invaluable role. They have provided critical support to airlift missions during numerous international emergencies including the Lebanon crisis (July–October of 1958), the Congo crisis (July–October of 1960), the Cuban crisis (September, 1962), the China–India confrontation (November, 1962–September, 1963), the Dominican Republic contingency and the Vietnam War, including the evacuation of Vietnam and Cambodia. CCTs were the last American unit to be evacuated from Khe Sahn on April 1, 1971.

From their involvement in Vietnam, the basis of modern Combat Control operating methods was formed, assuring mission safety, expediting air traffic flow and coordinating with local agencies and the airlift control element (ALCE).

It's the split-second reaction time of Combat Controllers that often make them the first on the scene as they were in Guatemala, Peru and Nicaragua after devastating earthquakes hit. Their humanitarian efforts have extended from helping the drought-stricken countries in North Africa to rescuing American hostages held in Iran in 1980.

Combat Controllers also held key roles in the success of other international military operations in the last two decades including the 1983 Grenada rescue operation, 1989 Panama Operation Just Cause, and both the pre-strike build-up of United Nations and American forces during Operation Desert Shield and the ensuing Desert Storm campaign.

The CCTs most recent success was in the struggle to capture Somalian leader Mohammed Fhara Aidid, during which a single Combat Controller, along with two PJs and several Army Rangers, was inserted into battle zone, established radio communications with gunship helos and provided direct fire calls to remove enemy threats, upon which the mission was completed and lives were saved.

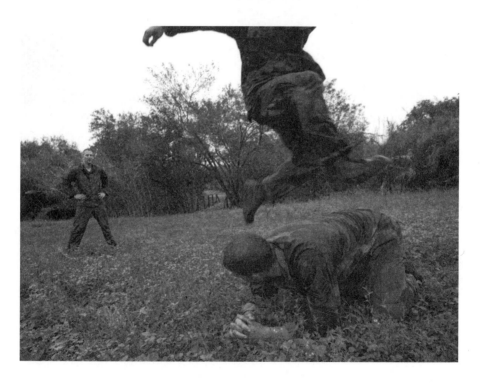

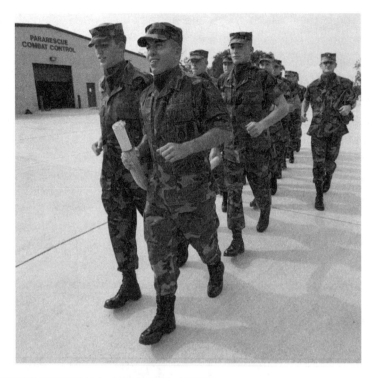

WHY BECOME A PJ OR CCT?

Aside from the incomparable distinction of being among the most highly trained and skilled specialists in the Air Force, recognized for your team's special operations capabilities and expertise, there are other noteworthy incentives to Pararescue and Combat Control. By completing Pararescue or Combat Control training, you have earned college credits with the Community College of the Air Force (CCAF). Additionally, technical and upgrade training is worth over 32 semester hours towards an Associates Degree in Applied Science or Survival and Rescue Operations. There is extensive travel as a Pararescueman or Combat Controller, requiring your aid in global missions supporting sister service components, allied forces, and humanitarian relief efforts, among other commitments. Both specialties receive additional incentive and/or specialty pays. And of course, you get to wear the distinctive beret according to your specialty, maroon for Pararescuemen and scarlet for Combat Controllers.

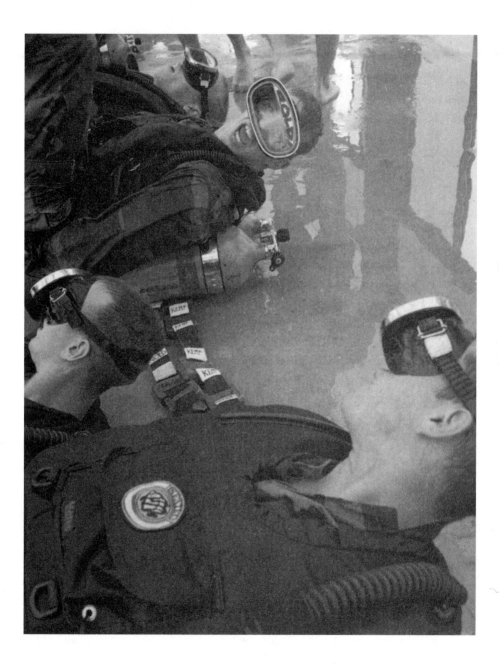

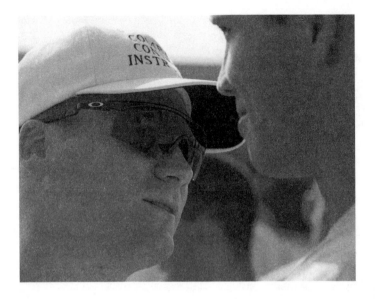

SO YOU WANT TO BE A PJ OR CCT?

Diving into choppy waters, jumping into thick jungle brush, or land-ing on an arctic glacier all require uniquely different physical and tech-nical expertise. The making of a PJ or a CCT consists of comprehensive training in a multitude of areas. Consequently, train-ing covers a wide range of deployment capabilities including the fol-lowing:

- Parachute operations in low/high altitudes (into forests, water)
- Waterborne infiltrations (SCUBA, aircraft boat drops, Rubber Raid-ing Craft operations, surface swimming)
- Mountain operations (Rock/ice climbing, rappelling, high angle evacuations)
- Helicopter operations (rappelling, fast rope, rope ladder, hoist operations, gunner/scanner)
- Overland movement (motorcycles, all-terrain vehicles, motor vehi-cles, team navigation)
- Arctic operations (cross-country skiing, downhill skiing, skijoring, snowmobiles, snowshoes, arctic sleds)

Total training lasts approximately 12–15 months and includes eight schools for each specialty. Normally students travel from school to school as a class, with the ranking student in charge. Training begins with the Pararescue/Combat Control Candidate Course.

THE PARARESCUE/COMBAT CONTROL CANDIDATE COURSE

Are you ready to carry out any assignment asked of you regardless of its apparent level of difficulty or threat to your own life? This is a question that must be considered before you take your first step into Pararescue or Combat Control Training. Both are jobs with extremely high demands requiring a dedication to training and personal sacrifice. What follows will give you a little taste of exactly what you and your body will commit to.

The Pararescue/Combat Control Candidate Course is where future PJs and CCTs are recruited, trained and selected. It is a highly structured and progressive ten-week course held in Lackland AFB, Texas,

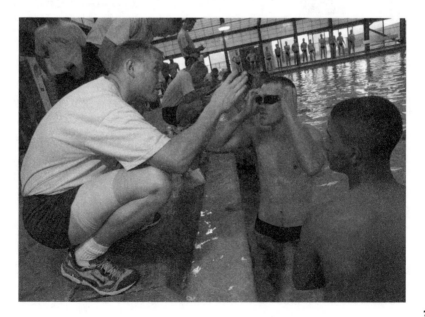

consisting of extensive and rigorous physical training and conditioning with swimming, running, weight training and calisthenics. It also includes physiological training, obstacle course, dive physics, metric manipulations, medical and dive terminology, CPR, weapons qualifications, history of PJs and CCT, and leadership laboratories. Once you

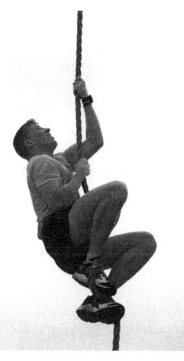

graduate from this course, you are not only fully prepared for the physical and mental demands of being a PJ or CCT, but you then move on to the "pipeline," training in more advanced specializations.

Training is broken down into two phases. Phase I, weeks 1-8, is known as team training, which focuses on teaching objective skills, progression of skills, building team unity, and preparation for the final course standards. Not only is the focus of this training on your ability to work together with your team but to prepare you for daily progress checks and weekly evaluations that you must pass in order to continue training. You receive instruction in metrics, medical and dive terminology and participate in four events daily of running, calisthenics, swimming, and water confidence exercises. Underwater training consists of underwater swim, mask and snorkel recovery, treading water, buddy breathing, drown proofing and weight belt swims, all of which help develop the much needed confidence when working underwater. Expect to be challenged physically and mentally like never before. One of Phase I's central goals is to develop your self-confidence and open your eyes to what you and your body are capable of accomplishing.

Weeks 9-10 comprise Phase II, called ancillary training, which entails M-9 weapons familiarization/qualification, CPR classes, physiological training and preparation for the pipeline.

TRAINING PIPELINE

Upon completion of the Candidate Course program, there are two different training pipelines to follow, depending upon what specialty you choose. You will learn extremely specialized skills to make you an expert in either Pararescue or Combat Control.

The Pararescue training track consists of the following specialty programs to prepare PJs for their work:

- **U.S. Army Airborne School – 3 weeks in Fort Benning, GA** This course takes personnel through basic parachuting skills after which they are awarded the basic parachutist rating and are allowed to wear the parachutist's wings.

- **U.S. Army Combat Divers School – 4 weeks in Key West, FL** This course provides training in SCUBA and becoming a combat diver, working to depths of 130 feet under various operating conditions.

- **U.S. Navy Underwater Egress Training – 1 day in Pensacola, FL** Training includes principles, procedures, and techniques necessary to escape from sinking aircraft.

- **U.S. Air Force Basic Survival School – 2.5 weeks in Fairchild, WA** Instruction in basic survival techniques including principles, procedures, and equipment. Enabling individuals to survive under various climates and environments is the central focus of this course.

- **U.S. Army Military Free-fall Parachutist School – 5 weeks in Ft. Bragg, NC and Yuma Proving Grounds, AZ** This more extensive course provides instruction and training in free-fall parachuting with a minimum of 30 free-fall jumps, including two day and two night jumps with supplemental oxygen and weight-bearing equipment.

- **Special Operations Combat Medic Course – 22 weeks in Fort Bragg, NC**   Phase I of this course consists of Emergency Medical Technician Basic (EMT-B) training. Phase II provides instruction in minor field surgery, pharmacology, trauma and airway management, and evacuation procedures. Upon graduating the course, you will be awarded with EMT-Paramedic certification through the National Registry.

- **Pararescue Recovery Specialist Course – 20 weeks in Kirtland, NM**   This course includes EMT-paramedic certification, field, mountaineering and combat tactics, advanced parachuting, helicopter, insertion and extraction techniques. This course qualifies airmen as Pararescue recovery specialists for any unit worldwide, after which they are awarded the maroon beret.

The Combat Control training track consists of several of the same advanced courses in addition to some exclusive training:

- **U.S. Army Airborne School**

- **U.S. Army Combat Divers School**

- **U.S. Air Force Basic Survival School**

- **U.S. Army Military Free-fall Parachutist School**

- **Combat Control Operator Course – 15.5 weeks in Keesler, MI**   This course provides instruction in aircraft recognition and performance, air navigation aids, weather, airport traffic control, flight assistance service, communication procedures, conventional approach control, radar procedures, and air traffic rules, all of which comprise the CCT's job.

- **Combat Control School – 12 weeks in Pope, NC**   Graduates receive final CCT qualifications, including land navigation, communications, assault zones, small unit tactics, parachute operations, and field tactics. Graduates are awarded the scarlet beret.

QUALIFICATIONS

In order to qualify for entry into the Candidate Course program, you must pass a physical entrance test called the Physical Abilities and Stamina Test (PAST). That means that your physical training needs to begin the moment you decide to enter the Candidate Course. The PAST consists of a series of exercises that must be completed in a specific order within a 3-hour time frame, with only a three-minute break between each exercise. Basically, you will

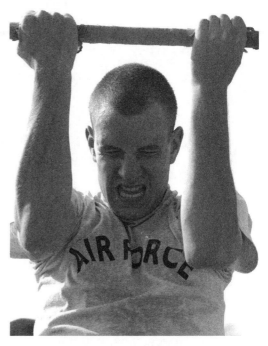

work your muscles to the point of exhaustion or until time has elapsed. Failure to meet any of the minimum standards means failure of the entire test and proper form is essential throughout.

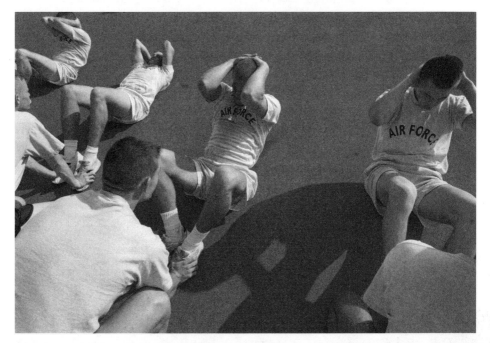

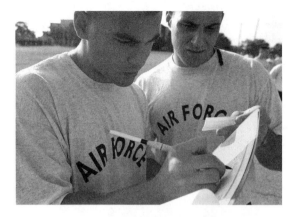

The PAST consists of the following:

Run 1.5 miles   in 10:30 minutes or less

Swim 1000 meters, side or
freestyle stroke,   in 26:00 minutes or less

Swim 25 meters
underwater without
resurfacing

Complete 8 chin-ups   in 1:00 minute or less

Complete 50 situps   in 2:00 minutes or less

Complete 50 pushups   in 2:00 minutes or less

Complete 50 flutter kicks   in 2:00 minutes or less

As mentioned, proper form is expected throughout. Therefore, it is critical that your body is trained ahead of time to not only guarantee that your muscles will perform, but so they will perform the right way.

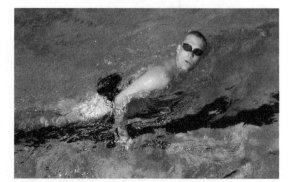

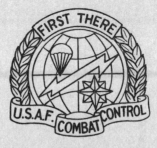

PART II:
FITNESS
TRAINING

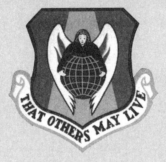

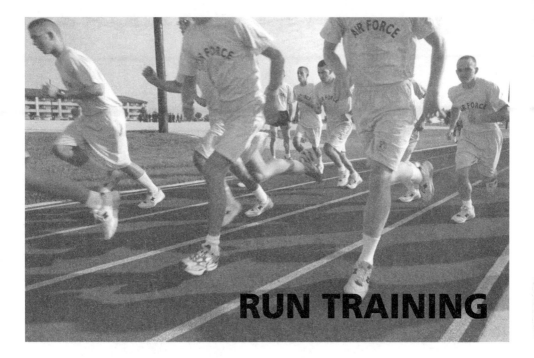

RUN TRAINING

If you cannot run three miles in under 21 minutes prior to the start of the Candidate Course, then you have some serious work ahead of you and a lot of mileage to cover. Pararescue and Combat Control training includes extensive running and rapid progression is expected. Lagging behind is not tolerated.

Regularity is critical in order to notice any improvement in your body's ability to run longer and farther. And you should know that a muscle begins to deteriorate if it's not worked in 72 hours. Also critical to your improvement is progression—your body will only continue to improve if the intensity of exercise is continually and gradually increased.

After several weeks of training, the duration of runs increases upwards of 50 minutes and your body had better be prepared to deliver speed and endurance. Preparation for run training should include three to four runs per week for 20 to 30 minutes, at a speed you can maintain without walking or stopping.

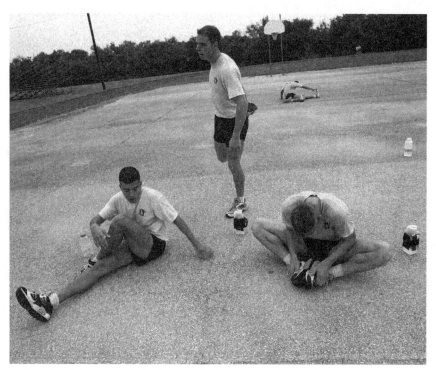

It is essential to stretch before and after running in order to minimize the chance of injury.

The various types of run training in the Candidate Course include long slow distance runs, fartlek runs, Indian sprints, and interval training. Evaluations take place on all-out distance running, covering as much ground in as short an amount of time as possible. The standard pace for an evaluated run is approximately a 7 to 7:10 minute mile, depending on the distance.

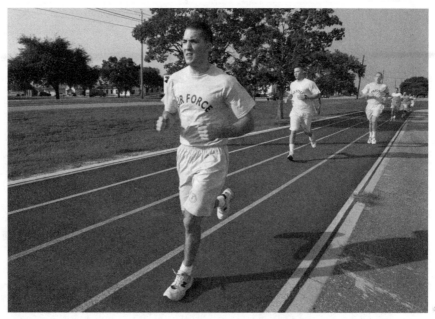

Stopping is not an option, no matter how tired you are!

MONITORING YOUR HEART RATE

Different types of running involve keeping track of your heart rate. Therefore, it is critical to understand and establish your Resting Heart Rate (RHR), Maximum Heart Rate (MHR), Maximum Heart Rate Reserve (MHRR) and Training Heart Rate (THR).

- *Your MHR is 220 minus your age*
- *Your MHHR equals your MHR minus RHR*
- *Your THR is established by multiplying MHRR by 60-90% (percentage depends upon run duration and level of fitness), then adding back your RHR*
- *Long Slow Distance running uses 60-75% MHRR*
- *Fartlek/ Last-man-up runs use 80-90% MHRR*
- *Interval runs use 75-90% MHRR*
- *Race pace (evaluations) runs use 95-100% MHRR*

43

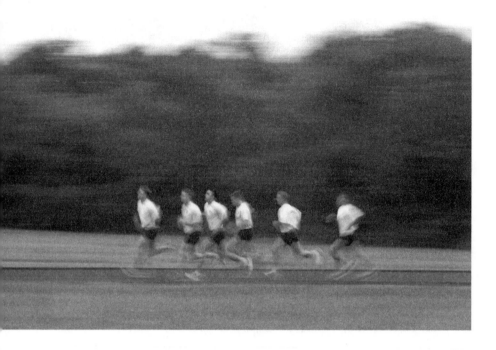

LONG SLOW DISTANCE RUNS

Its name says it all—long, slow, and covering lots of distance. The pace for LSD is set by the instructor and is normally equivalent to 60-75% of the students' MHRR. LSD helps build cardiovascular strength and endurance and facilitates efficient oxygen transfer in the body.

- The warm-up consists of 20 minutes of stretching and 5 minutes of light jogging before the pace is set.

- Depending on the size of the team, there are normally three different run groups according to ability.

- Style and performance are critiqued during and after each run with particular attention paid to effort and teamwork, a lack of which may result in additional time added to the run or supplemental calisthenics.

- A cool down jog for 5 to 10 minutes concludes the run and is followed by 20 minutes of stretching, after debriefing.

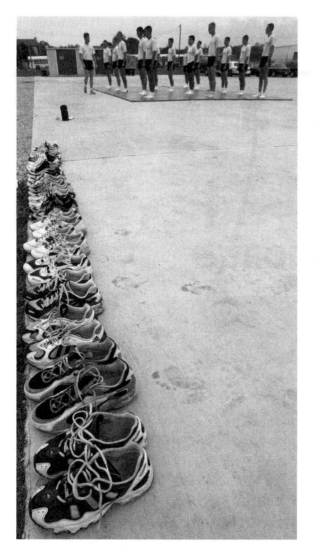

Proper running shoes are crucial to avoiding injuries. PJ/CCT trainees are permitted to choose the very best footwear suited for their running style and foot shape, rather than being issued a standard "one size fits most" athletic shoe as is common with most military training units.

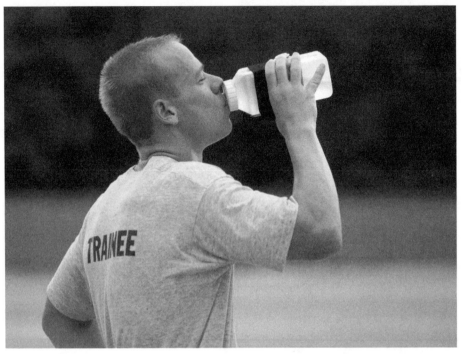

Drink plenty of water before, during, and after exercise. Dehydration can be a PJ/CCT trainee's worst enemy!

INTERVAL RUNS

Regardless of how tired you are, interval training is all about constant speed. Work intervals use 75-90% MHRR. In order to build up speed and pace, you'll run faster than the previous week's evaluation.

- The warm-up consists of 12 minutes of jogging and 20 minutes of stretching before beginning the interval work.

- Rest periods between intervals allow for students to concentrate on lowering heart rate and preparing for the next interval.

- Instructors critique style and performance following each interval. Students should be within one second above pace or two seconds below it. If not, they will be moved into another interval group.

- The cool-down consists of 10 to 12 minutes of jogging and 20 minutes of stretching after the training ends.

FARTLEK RUNS

Fartlek training is also known as "last man up" and the key to it is constant speed during the fast portion of the run. This training usually takes place on long flat terrain, hills, or a mixture of both. Work intervals (the fast portions) use 80-90% MHRR. Though it may mean going all out, pushing beyond the previous week's evaluation pace is what will build up speed and leg strength. Again, careful attention is paid to the effort exerted by students who are expected to keep up with the pace and put forth maximum effort.

- The warm-up consists of a five minute run and 20 minutes of stretching before setting the pace.

- Instructors normally run four minutes hard, then slow down the heart rate to 80-85%, until the scheduled time has elapsed.

- The 10 minute cool-down begins after total time has elapsed. After debriefing, students stretch for 20 minutes.

TRAINING RUNS

Training runs take place on varied types of terrain. The lead instructor may opt to alter the running path in order to introduce the students to running on off-road terrain. Aside from building balance and coordination, running on different terrain more closely mirrors what students will encounter in the line of duty. Some examples of different types of training runs include:

- Running under tree branches, logs, or small obstacles

- Hopping over logs, small fences, or obstacles

- Running/walking through dense woods

- Running/walking up or down steep wooded hills

- Crossing creeks no higher than waist deep

- Fording creeks chest high, no more than 50 yards at a time

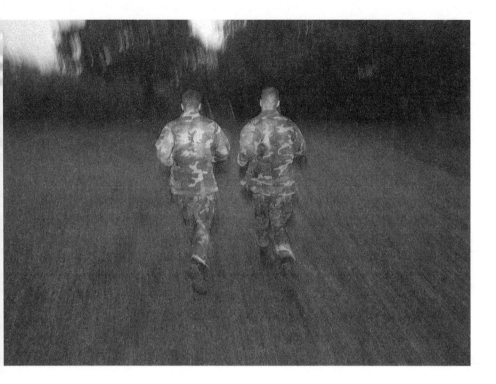

- Running through creeks, no deeper than knee high
- Low or high crawling short distances, no more than 50 yards at a time, continuing with a run
- Log roll down hills (to experience sensory deprivation), then running up the hill

WATER CONFIDENCE AND SWIM TRAINING

Swimming is a large part of Candidate Course training. Typically, a trainee will swim 2000 meters or more in a training session. That means your body better be prepared for the underwater rigors that await. Prior to beginning training, a candidate should swim 1500 to 2000 meters, three to five times per week, with the intention of being capable of swimming 1500 meters using freestyle or side stroke in under 45 minutes.

Hold your breath—underwater swimming (that means swimming distances under water without surfacing) is another element of training. Prior to graduation a trainee must successfully complete a 50-meter underwater swim. The better you become at underwater swimming, the more prepared your body will be to handle the evaluated tasks and SCUBA requirements that the Candidate Course has in store for you.

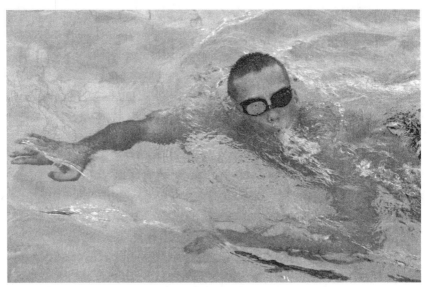

Good form includes proper breathing techniques.

FORM

Freestyle swimming is used frequently throughout swim training. Proper body position is referred to as the prone position, straight and nearly horizontal but just below the surface of the water. The head should be aligned with the body, with the waterline at the hairline. The natural roll that the head and body have during the swim stroke helps to allow for maximum propulsion by the arms, effective inhalation, and easy recovery. The legs work to propel with a flutter kick originating from the hip. (More effective forward propulsion results from relaxed ankles and feet.) The legs also serve as a rudder to guide the body through the water. For extra speed, swimmers can use a narrow kick about the width of the body. This kick is initiated at the knee, causing a whipping action of the feet.

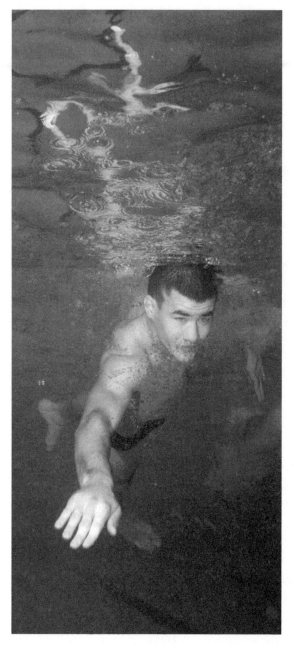

BREATHING

Your head should remain in line with your spine throughout the swim stroke. When the arm on the breathing side of the body is about one-half to three-quarters of the way through its backward pressing action, the head should rotate independently with the use of the shoulders. While inhaling, the cheek opposite to the breathing side should remain flat to the water. Exhalation should occur through the mouth and continue until the next inhalation. Inhalation and exhalation occur in every stroke. Alternating breathing sides is best for a balanced stroke.

TECHNIQUE

To coordinate the arm action of a swim stroke, the hand must enter the water forward of the shoulder, fingertips first, thumb side of the hand rotated downward slightly, and the elbow bent and held higher than the hand. The opposite arm should be halfway through its pressing action, with the elbow bent and hand under the midline of the body. This arm should be accelerating to complete the pressing action. The entry hand slides forward and downward until fully extended. When at this point, the opposite arm has almost completed its backward pressing action and inhalation is just about complete. From the extended position, the entry arm and hand begin to pull backward toward the center of the body. The elbow is always kept higher than the hand and lower than the shoulder during propulsion movements. The opposite arm begins to recover when the forward arm starts to pull. Upon finishing the backward thrust of the arm on the breathing side, the elbow is immediately lifted up and out of the water with continued momentum. The body and shoulders should roll easily to help arm recovery and propulsion. During recovery, the lower hand pulls backward with the bend at the elbow increasing. The elbow should be bent to its maximum when the lower arm and hand are pressed back below and in front of the shoulder.

Maintain an open palm during the entire backward push. At this point, the opposite arm is about halfway through recovery and the lower arm should begin to accelerate the backward pressing action. As the hand enters the water, the head and body begin the rolling action onto the side of the entry arm and the arm actions take place on the opposite sides of the body.

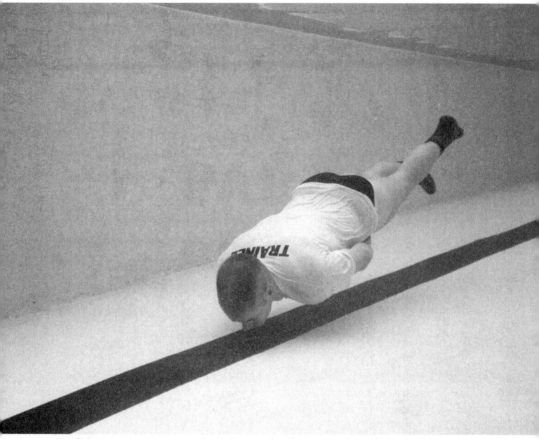

Candidates sometimes train using only their arms or legs to increase strength and improve technique.

UNDERWATER SWIMMING

Underwater swimming is simply a modified breaststroke, where the arm pulls down farther toward the rear for more thrust through the water. A dive mask is worn throughout. During a training session, students line up at one end of the pool and wait for the instructor to initiate the exercise. On command, students swim from one end of the pool (approximately 25 meters) to the other end without surfacing. Once they touch the opposite wall, they swim a freestyle sprint back to the starting point as fast as they can. The exercise is repeated until the required number of underwater exercises has been completed.

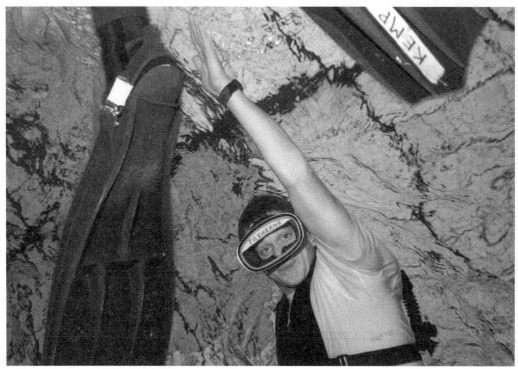

All evaluated swims are performed with fins.

FIN SWIMMING

All of the swims evaluated in the Candidate Course are distance swims in which students wear "rocket" style fins. During fin swimming, the swimmer holds a prone glide position, keeping one arm locked out in front of the body to guide the body in the intended direction. The other arm either trails behind or propels in a sidestroke. Although legs are used to flutter kick for propulsion, knees should remain locked with all movement originating at the hip. Kicks are performed with the knees locked and toes pointed. Breathing is similar to that in freestyle swimming but takes place on one side only, that being the one opposite to the extended arm.

During the fin swimming exercise, in addition to rocket style fins, swimmers wear dive masks, booties and a T-shirt. The exercise begins

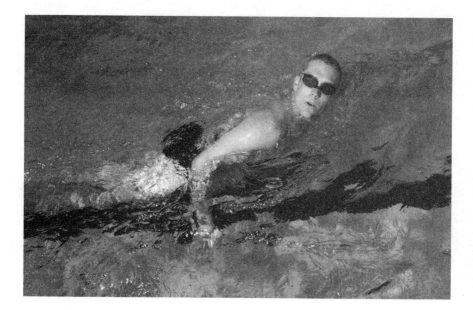

with each student in a swim lane against the wall. On command, students leave the wall and begin to swim using a flutter kick to propel them down the lane. Swimming should be done on the side or stomach only, with one arm extended out and ahead of the body. Students turn at the opposite end of the pool and continue to swim the required number of laps. No freestyle strokes or dolphin kicks are allowed during fin swimming. Students may also be asked to do sprints, during which they must sprint-swim as quickly as possible. This is followed by a rest period before the next sprint. Swimming exercises are considered successfully completed when they are done in the correct manner within a prescribed time period.

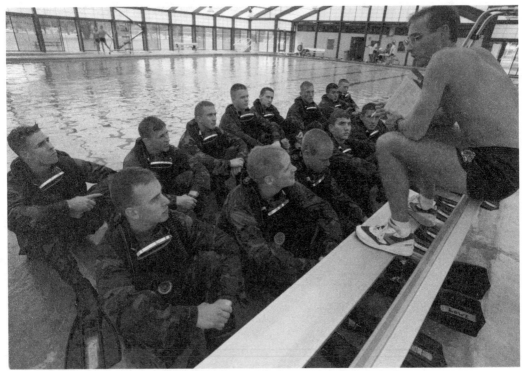

Students are briefed and evaluated before and after each swim period.

WATER CONFIDENCE TRAINING

Water confidence training is meant to do exactly that—build your confidence in the water, increase the amount of time you can spend underwater, and better your handling of high-stress situations. There are a number of pool training events during which students are evaluated. The following training events describe activities that can threaten safety, possibly leading to "shallow water blackout," brain damage or death. **Do not perform these exercises unless there is a lifeguard within close proximity.**

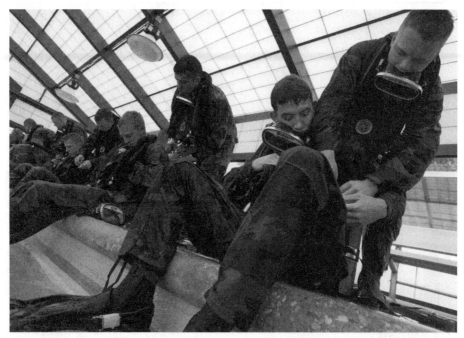

Students help prepare teammates before water confidence exercises.

Mask and Snorkel Recovery. This exercise begins with all students at one end of the pool. The instructor throws or places a student's mask and snorkel a specified distance from him. On the command "Go," the student swims underwater to his mask and snorkel. Upon reaching them, he is to place the snorkel between his knees and position the mask on his face, clearing it of water. The student than ascends to the surface with the snorkel in his mouth and left arm extended above his head with a clenched fist. Successful completion of the exercise is indicated by a clear mask and snorkel, allowing for adequate vision and breathing.

Buddy Breathing/Pool Harassment. In the deep end of the pool, on command, students place their faces into the water and begin to survival float while buddy breathing from one snorkel. One hand maintains control of the student; the other passes the snorkel. Students are only allowed to breathe through the snorkel, never lifting their heads from the water. Completion of this exercise entails

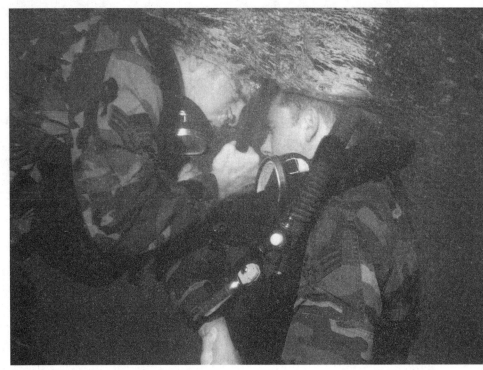

Buddy breathing.

keeping the head in the water, remaining calm, and maintaining control of the buddy and snorkel for the designated time. Pool harassment is a more intense form of buddy breathing. It involves the instructor entering the water and provoking students with stressful situations, trying to incite a panic reaction.

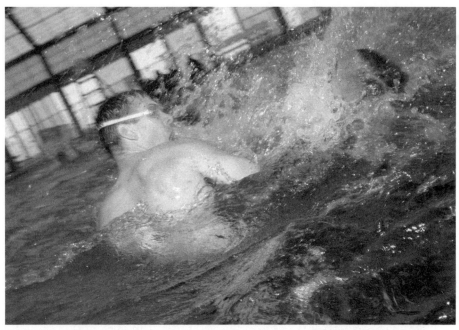

Pool harassment: Instructors try to provoke students with stressful situations in order to test their confidence and ability to remain calm.

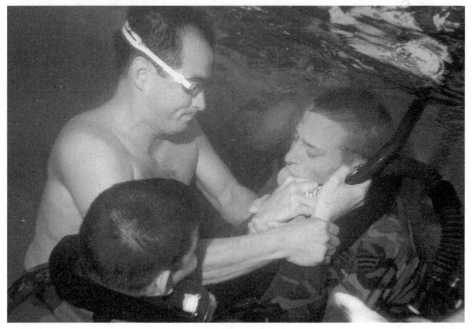

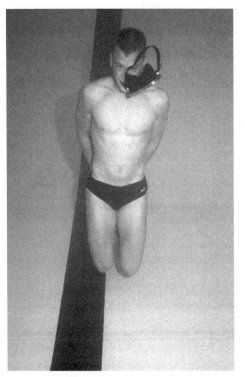

Drownproofing: Mask recovery.

Drownproofing. This exercise is accomplished through four tasks, with students divided into pairs, one acting as a safety monitor. The student's hands and feet are bound as he stands on the deck in the deep end of the pool, before being tapped into the water.

The first task is *bobbing*, where the student sinks to the bottom of the pool and then pushes off, exhaling until reaching the surface. Upon reaching the surface, the student inhales and repeats the process.

The second task is *floating*. The student inhales as much air as possible, tucks the chin into the chest, bends forward at the waist, and relaxes, staying within a 4 x 4-meter square. The head is brought out of the water to inhale, then brought back to float position.

The third task is *traveling*. Students dolphin kick 100 meters without touching the bottom or sides of the pool, using the feet and knees to propel them through the water.

The fourth task consists of *flips* and *mask recovery*. After traveling, the student begins bobbing again. Within five bobs the student performs a front flip underwater, then within five more bobs performs a backward flip. A mask is then thrown to the bottom of the pool, after which the student must swim and retrieve it with his teeth, and then complete five more bobs.

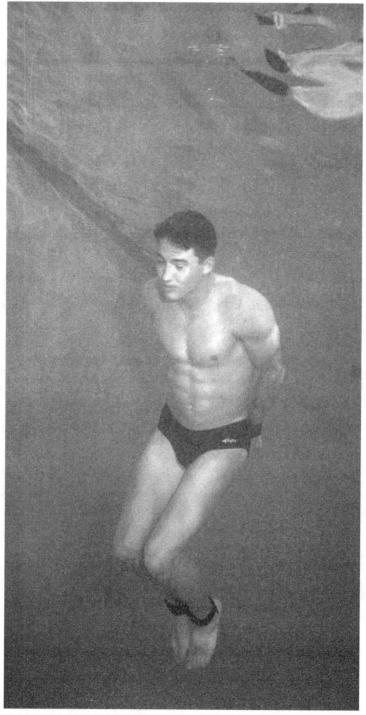

Drownproofing: Bobbing.

Lifesaving. In this exercise, one student acts as a victim and the other performs the rescue. Students are evaluated on two water entries, the long shallow dive and the stride jump; two basic lifesaving rescues—front surface approach to an inactive victim and underwater approach to an active victim; and three releases (when the victim grabs the rescuer, the rescuer must free himself in order to save the victim)—the double grip on one wrist release, the front head hold release and the rear head hold release.

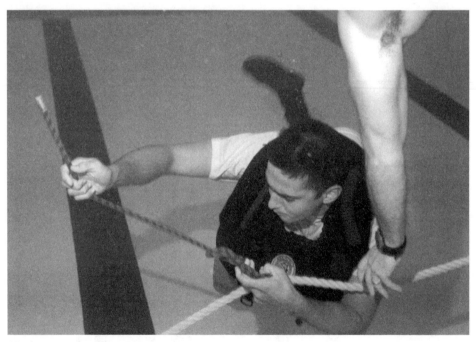

Underwater knots.

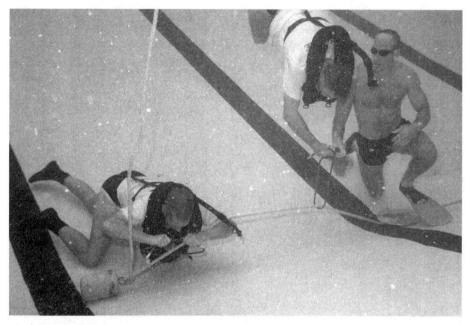

Underwater knots.

Underwater Knots. The knots taught in this exercise are the bow-line, square knot, and girth hitch. Students spread out over the length of an underwater rope treading water. Each student has two ropes, one in hand, the other in their trunks. On command, students descend to the underwater rope and tie the designated knot prior to surfacing. Knots must be tied properly, dressed with their tails no less than four inches.

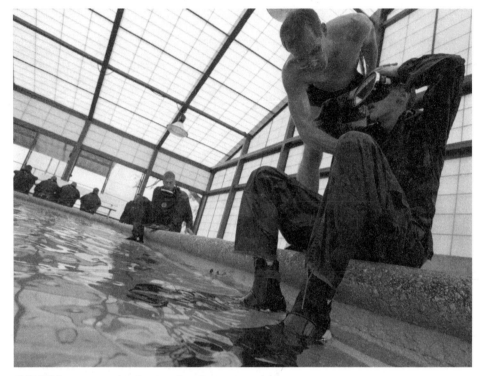

INDOC instructor checks a trainee's gear poolside.

Ditch and Donning. Students begin this exercise lined up facing the deep end of the pool, wearing masks, fins, booties, a t-shirt and a weighted belt. On command they begin treading water, while moving to the deep end. On command, students make a clear water surface dive to the deepest part of the pool and ditch their gear, placing each piece of equipment in a very specific manner, and then ascending to the top. On command, they dive to retrieve their gear, again in a particular sequential order. They must then clear their mask, ascend to the surface, and exit the water with hands on top of their heads, to await judgement on their performance.

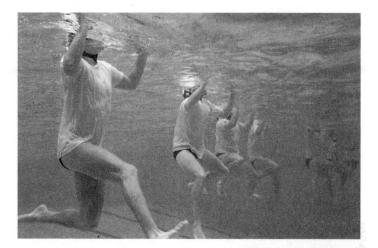

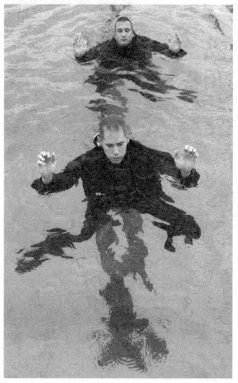

Treading Water. In deep water, students attempt to tread water with their hands raised above their heads, using only their legs. Correct form requires keeping your hands and head above the water, using your legs in an egg-beater kicking motion, both rhythmical and forceful enough to maintain adequate buoyancy.

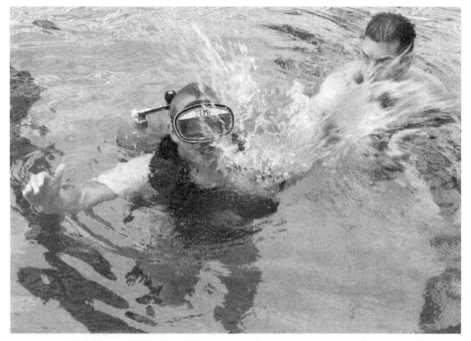

PJ/CCT trainee treads water with SCUBA tanks while the instructor provides "harassment".

Weight Belt Swim. Also in the deep end of the pool, students must swim continuously on their side with a leading arm out in front for a designated time period, all the while wearing full gear and a sixteen-pound weight belt. The student must swim on the side they choose first, without switching, for the entire time.

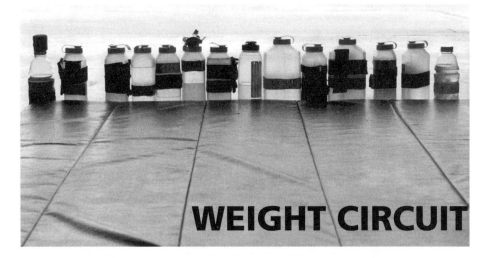

WEIGHT CIRCUIT

Muscular fitness is a combination of strength (the ability to exert force) and endurance (the ability to exert force over a sustained amount of time).

Because weight training is essential to building muscular fitness, it is a core component of the Pararescue/Combat Control Candidate Course. The principles of muscular training are based on the following:

The major muscle groups to be worked include:
Legs: quadriceps, hamstrings, and gluteals
Chest: pectorals, triceps, and deltoids
Back: latissimus dorsi, biceps, and rhomboids
Shoulders: deltoids and triceps

- Overload—Giving the muscle more than it's used to
- Progression—Increasing weight over a steady period of time
- Specificity—Precision when working a specific muscle
- Regularity—Training on a regular basis
- Recovery—Giving the muscle adequate time to recover between work periods

- Balance—Working muscles equally, not one more than another
- Variety—Performing a variety of different exercises on a muscle

For a muscle to become stronger, it needs to be worked more strenuously. As the workload increases, the muscle must adapt by becoming stronger and larger—this is the basis of the overload principle. An effective weight training program incorporates methods including increasing resistance, increasing the number of repetitions per set, increasing the number of sets, and reducing the rest time between sets.

During the Candidate Course, weight training is scheduled twice a week using a "circuit training" technique, which requires students to complete a series of exercises at a specified pace for a fixed duration.

How to find your 1RM

(Resistance Measure)

1. *Warm up with a weight with which you can do 10-15 repetitions.*

2. *After a three to five minute rest, try to lift your perceived 1RM.*

3. *If you can lift the weight three or more times, take another rest, and try to lift with 10% more weight added to your perceived 1RM.*

4. *If this weight is too heavy, subtract 10% and try again after resting.*

5. *If you can only do one rep with a specific weight then that is your 1RM.*

Before beginning your weight training program, you should determine the resistance (the amount of weight) appropriate for your level. To do this, you need to establish what is called your 1RM, or resistance measure (see inset).

Keep in mind that you should adhere to standard phases of conditioning muscles for the maximum response:

Preparatory phase—Using lighter weights during the first week of training is conducive to developing proper lifting technique, form, and breathing, as well as reducing the chances of injury.

Conditioning phase—As muscular strength and endurance increase, the intensity of the workout, including the amount of weight used, should increase simultaneously. When 12 or more reptitions feel comfortable, it's time to add some weight to your program (but do not exceed 10% of the original weight).

Maintenance phase—Once a high level of fitness has been achieved, maintenance becomes the important factor. Shift the focus from progression to retention.

The USAF Elite Weight Circuit Training Program:

Weeks 1-2: One circuit of each exercise, exercising for 30 seconds, 15 repetitions at 60% of your 1RM, then a 30-second rest and switch to the next station.

Weeks 3-5: Two circuits of each exercise, exercising for 30 seconds, 15 repetitions at 60% of your 1RM, then a 30-second rest and switch to the next station.

Weeks 6-8: Three circuits of each exercise, exercising for 30 seconds, 15 reps at 60% of your 1RM, then a 30-second rest and switch to the next station.

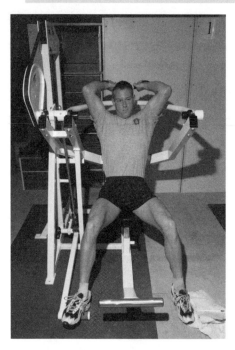 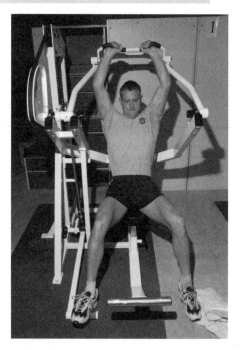

STATION 1   TRICEPS MACHINE

Muscles Worked: *Triceps*

While seated, reach back and grasp the bar, palms facing upward. Lift the weight just above your head, in a smooth and continuous motion. Gently lower the weight—this is called the "negative" movement.

Be sure to warm up before your workout, especially before determining your 1RM. An ideal warm-up should consist of five to ten minutes of brisk walking or light jogging.

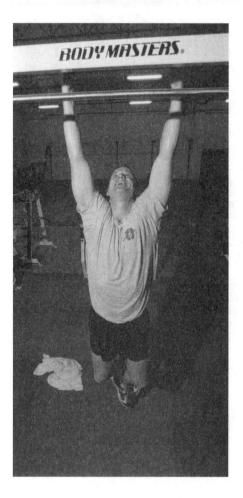

STATION 2   PULL-UPS

Muscles Worked: *Latissimus Dorsi, Biceps, Forearms*

Pull-ups are an important part of weight circuit training. Here the weight is you—and lifting your own body weight is a great way to build your back and arms.

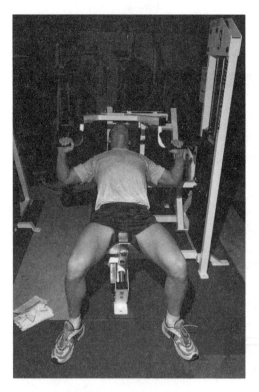
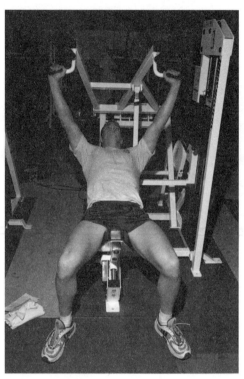

STATION 3 INCLINE CHEST

Muscles Worked: *Upper Pectorals, Anterior Deltoid, Triceps*
Laying on your back, grasp the bar, palms facing upward. In a slow
and steady motion, lift the weight straight up. Bring the weight
down in the same slow and controlled motion.

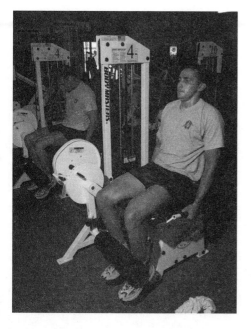

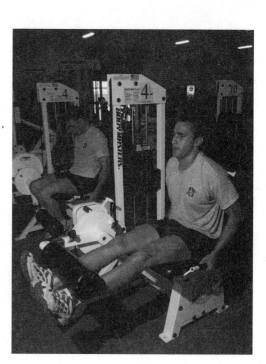

STATION 4   LEG EXTENSION

Muscles Worked: *Quadriceps*

While sitting, slide your legs underneath the lifting bar. The pads should be resting comfortably on your ankles. Lift the weight upward and outward until your leg is straight, providing a full contraction of the quadriceps muscle. Your toes should be pointing upward.

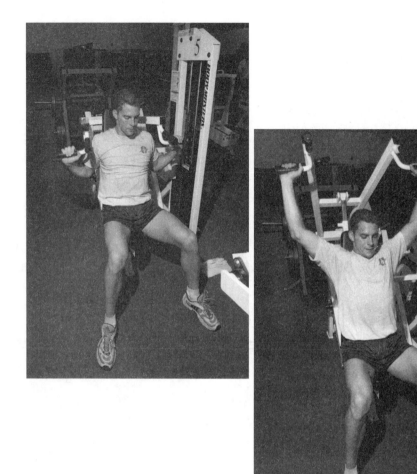

STATION 5   MILITARY PRESS

Muscles Worked: *Deltoid, Triceps*

While seated, grasp the bar with your palms facing outward. Lift the weight in a vertical movement, from shoulder height to full extension—though locking your elbows is not necessary.

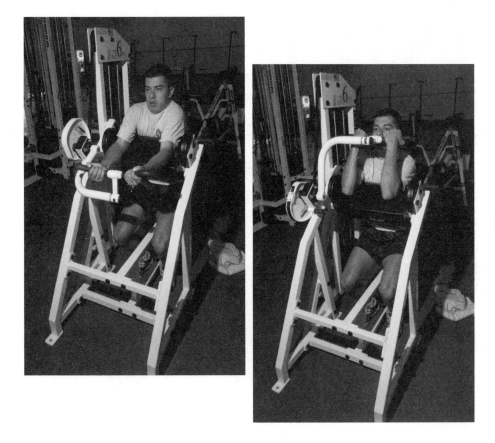

STATION 6   BICEPS CURL

Muscles Worked: *Biceps*

Grasp the weight with the palms up and slightly facing toward you. Making sure to keep your elbows in, lift the weight up and toward your chin, providing a full contraction of the biceps muscle at the top of the motion.

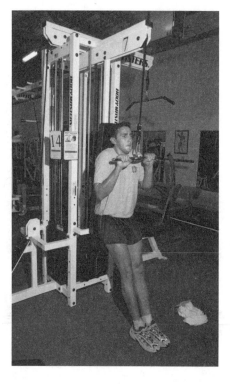
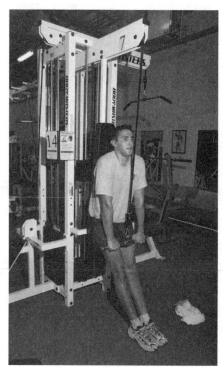

STATION 7   TRI-PUSHDOWN

Muscles Worked: *Triceps*

Grasp the weight in front of you, shoulder high, palms facing out. Keeping your elbows in at all times, press the bar down until your elbows are locked, providing a full contraction of the triceps. Make sure to perform this exercise in a smooth and continuous motion for maximum benefit.

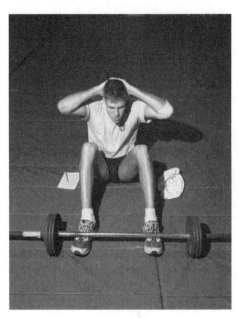

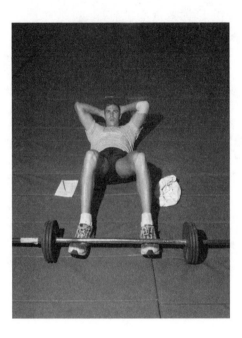

STATION 8 SITUPS

Muscles Worked: *Abdominal*

Though not a weight lifting exercise per se, situps (and crunches) are included in the circuit course for two reasons: 1) to provide a "break" to allow for your muscles to recover and 2) because you can never do too many! Keep your hands behind your head but do not lift with your hands! This can cause a neck strain. Do them right!

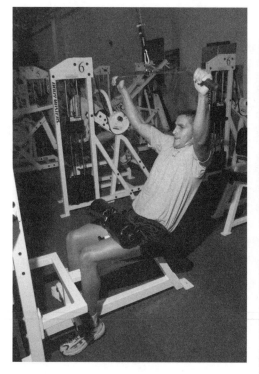
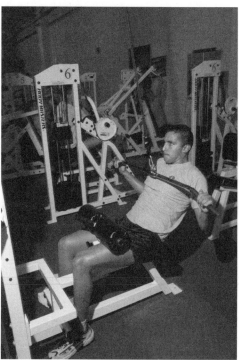

STATION 9   PULL DOWN

Muscles Worked: *Latissimus Dorsi, Posterior Deltoid, Forearms*
Grasp the bar, palms facing outward. Pull the weight down to your chest. Try to squeeze your elbows together behind your back in order to maximize the effect of this station.

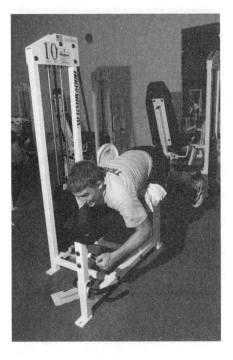
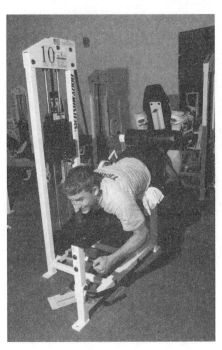

STATION 10   LEG CURLS

Muscles Worked: *Hamstrings*

Laying face down, place the back of your ankles—not your calves—behind the padded lifting bar. Your ankles should be comfortable, without pain. Grab the hand grips below the bench and slowly lift your legs, bending the knees, trying to touch your ankles to your buttocks.

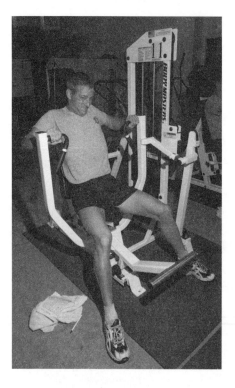
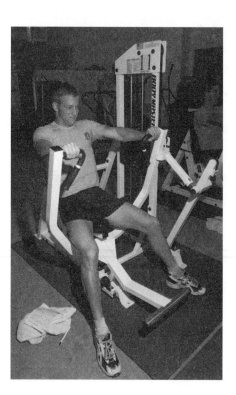

STATION 11   CHEST PRESS

Muscles Worked: *Pectorals, Anterior Deltoid, Triceps*

Adjust the seat so the handles are in line with your chest and shoulder upon full extension. Push the weight slowly away from you until your arms are fully extended. Return to the starting position and repeat—feel the burn in your chest muscles!

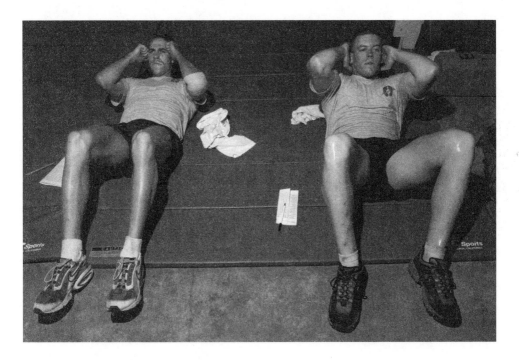

STATION 12   CRUNCHES

Muscles Worked: *Upper Abdominal*

Work those abs again! Proper technique is required to reduce the chances of injury. Feel the exercise in your abs alone—no cheating with your neck or back.

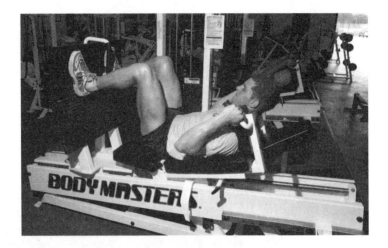

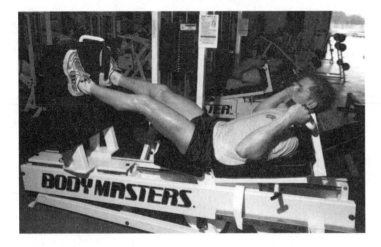

STATION 13   LEG PRESS

Muscles Worked: *Quadriceps, Gluteals, Hamstrings*

Place your feet flat against the press panel as shown. Grab the handles by the side of your head and slowly push away from the panel in a smooth motion until your legs are fully extended—without locking your knees! Return the weight to the starting position in a controlled motion in order to minimize the amount of stress on your knees.

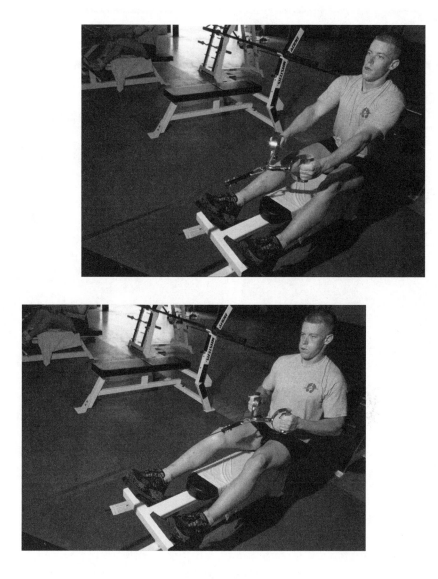

STATION 14   SEATED ROWS

Muscles Worked: *Latissimus Dorsi, Biceps, Forearms*
As the name implies, this machine mimics the movement of rowing a boat. Keep you elbows tucked in close to your sides and your lower back arched. This will help avoid potential lower back stress injuries.

83

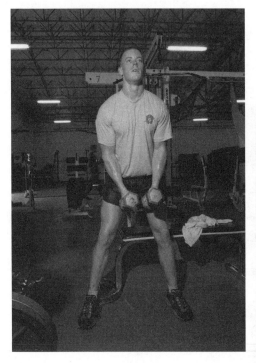

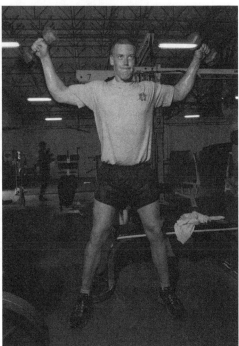

STATION 15   LAT RAISES

Muscles Worked: *Deltoids*

Use free weights for this one. Start with the weights in the "down" position as shown. Slowly lift the weights over your shoulders, then return to the down position. Repeat.

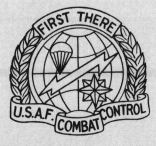

PART III: WORK OUT WITH THE USAF ELITE

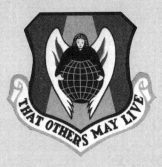

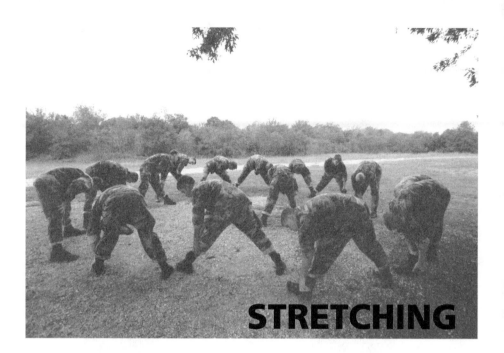

STRETCHING

In addtion to strength and endurance, you need flexibility to help you move your joints through a full range of motion. Logically speaking, limber muscles can stretch farther and work longer than stiff, inflexible ones. All workouts must include a warm-up and cool down period that include stretching exercises to help develop flexibility and prevent injury. Some important stretching guidelines:

- Always warm up the body with some type of light aerobic activity such as jumping jacks prior to stretching.
- Stretches should be performed slowly and held in position—jerky movements are futile and can cause injury.
- Stretches should be held between 15 seconds and 2 minutes—the longer you hold a stretch, the more it will help increase flexibility.

87

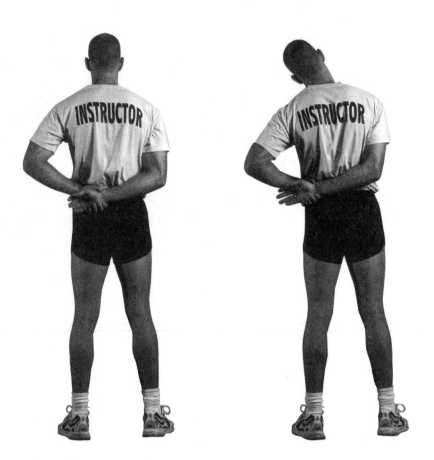

NECK STRETCH

This is an excellent stretch for both the neck and shoulders. Tilt your head to the left while gently pulling your right arm across your back as shown. Feel the stretch on the top of your shoulder and into your neck. Repeat on the opposite side.

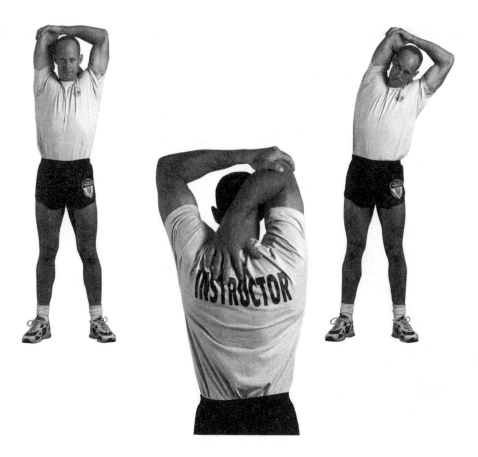

TRICEPS STRETCH

Pull your right arm behind your head and reach down toward the middle of your shoulder blades as shown. You can pull on your right arm gently for added stretch. Lean to the left to add some stretch to your lats. Repeat on the opposite side.

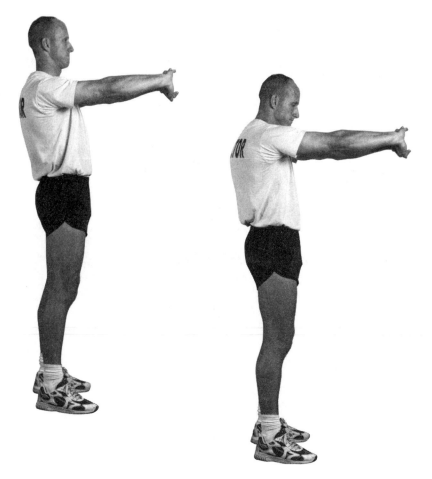

MIDDLE BACK STRETCH

Lace your fingers together while reaching forward as shown. Roll your shoulders forward as you stretch your shoulder blades and back. Feel good? It should!

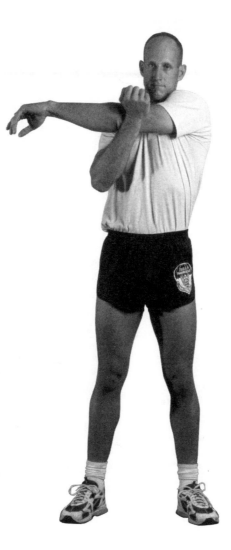

SHOULDER STRETCH

Extend your left arm across your chest. Place your right hand behind your left elbow as shown. Keeping your shoulders level (don't drop your left arm!), squeeze and pull your extended arm with the other hand, stretching your shoulder muscles, the deltoids.

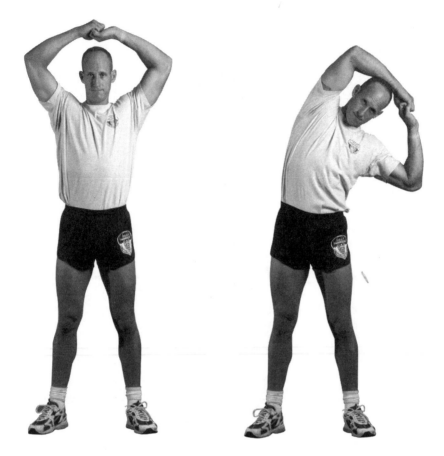

SIDE STRETCH

With your feet shoulder width apart, grasp your hands above your head, keeping your elbows bent. As you lean to the left, pull with your left hand. Keep your knees "soft." In other words, slightly bend your knees to avoid putting pressure on them and risking injury. Return to the starting position and lean to the right, pulling with your right hand.

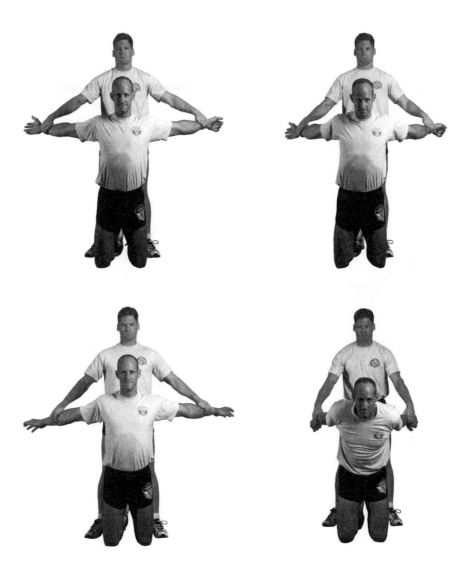

TWO-MAN CHEST STRETCH WITH DELTOID VARIATION

For this stretch, you'll need a workout partner. With your partner behind you, kneel on the floor and extend your arms to the side, keeping them level with your shoulders. With your chest "proud" (and you should be proud!) allow your partner to easily pull your arms behind you, so you feel the stretch in your chest muscles, the pectorals.

> If you have trouble keep-
> ing your balence, grab a
> door or lean on a buddy's
> shoulder. Eventually you'll
> be able to do this stretch
> without assistance.

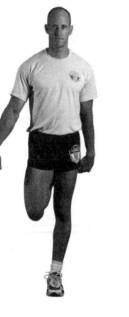
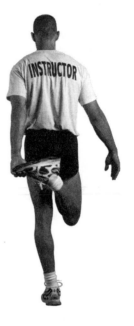

STANDING QUAD STRETCH

This stretch targets the muscles in the front of your thighs, the quadriceps. Standing on your left leg, bend your right leg at the knee and
lift it behind your back. Grabbing your right ankle with your left hand,
gently pull behind and across, while you stretch your quads. Repeat
on the opposite side.

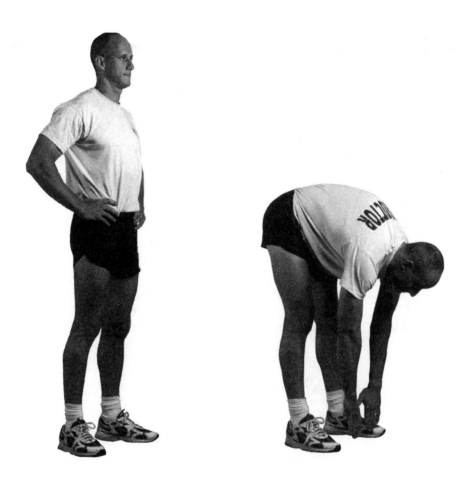

STANDING HAMSTRING STRETCH

Start with your hands on your hips. Bend at the waist, reaching to touch your toes. Keep your legs straight, or just slightly bent if you are a beginner. You should feel the stretch in the back of your legs, not in your lower back! Keep your back straight as you bend down, and try to bend down as far as you can. If you can't reach the floor, that's okay. Give it some time.

If you bend your rear knee and lift your rear heel, you'll feel the stretch in your Achilles tendon. Why not try it!

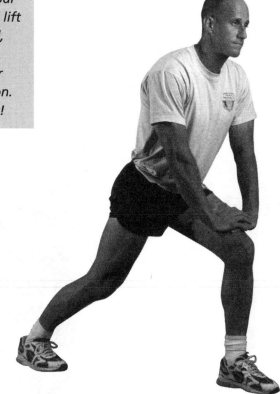

STANDING CALF STRETCH

Take a step forward with your left leg. Keep your toes pointed straight ahead, as shown. Placing your hands on your forward knee, lean forward while keeping your rear foot firmly planted and rear leg fairly straight. Do not lift your heel. Feel the stretch run up the back of your lower leg. Switch sides and repeat.

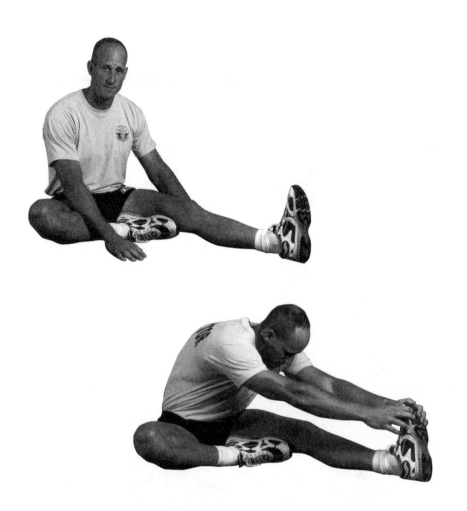

MODIFIED HURDLER STRETCH

Sitting on the floor, bring your foot in toward your upper thigh as shown in the photo. This stretches your back and hamstrings. Reach out for your toes. Come on, you can reach them! Repeat with the opposite leg.

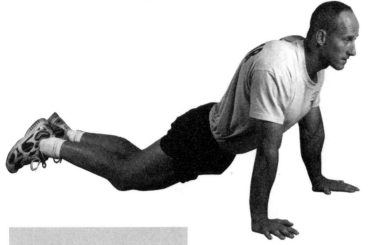

This stretch is great for the abs, but you want to make certain not to overstretch! Do not apply excess pressure as you perform the cobra. You can injure your lower back.

THE COBRA STRETCH

This stretch takes its name from the image of the deadly cobra snake as it is poised to strike. Take a position on the floor with your knees down and your body supported by your outstretched arms. Gently— repeat gently—press your hips downward toward the floor, feeling the stretch in your abs.

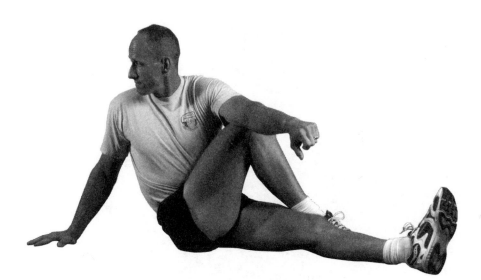

LOWER BACK STRETCH

This is a great hip and back stretch, and helps stretch your ITB, or ili-otibial band. Sitting down, cross your right leg over your left, as shown in the photo. Now gently twist your torso to the right, press-ing your left arm against your right leg. Repeat on the opposite side.

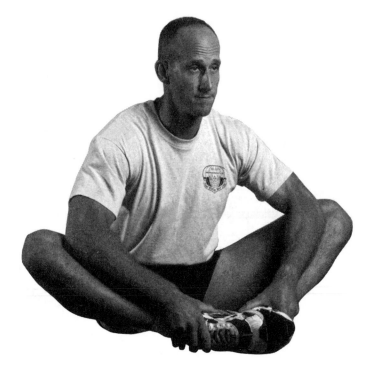

BUTTERFLY STRETCH

This stretches the groin muscles. Tuck your heels in towards your groin. Try to bring your knees to the floor by pushing down with your elbows.

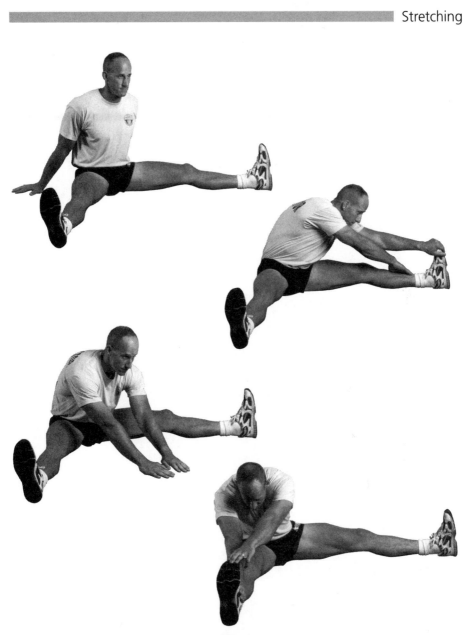

MODIFIED BUTTERFLY STRETCH

Start with legs spread wide apart. Now lean to touch your left toes. Come up, then lean forward to touch the floor between your legs. Come to the starting position once more, and then lean to touch your right toes. Great for the legs, groin, and lower back muscles. Just make sure you don't rush and don't bounce—your movements should be smooth.

101

UPPER BODY EXERCISES

Pushups—and their many variations—are a standard exercise performed during basic military training. You will do a lot of these at the Candidate Course, without a doubt! The most important thing to remember when doing upper body exercises is to maintain proper form—back straight, eyes forward . . . and one and two, . . .

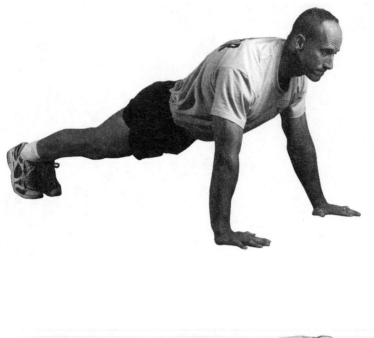

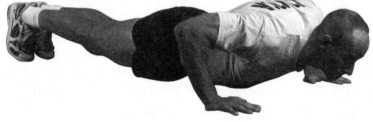

STANDARD PUSHUP

The classic exercise of all military fitness training regimens! Not only a great upper body exercise, pushups (or the threat of doing them) can be great motivators! Back straight and eyes forward, arms about shoulder width apart. Lower yourself in a controlled fashion. Don't let your chest touch the ground. Return to the starting position.

Your ability to perform pushups is an important part of the PAST. Plus, be prepared to do many of these during your INDOC course!

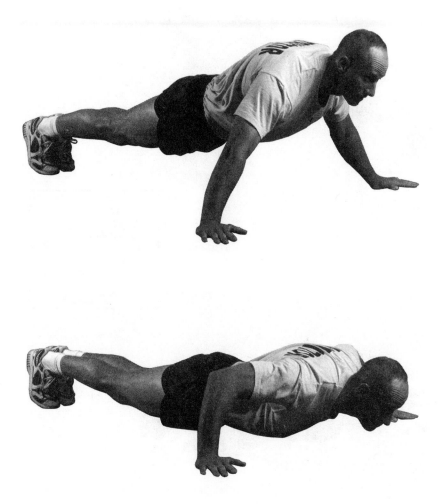

WIDE STANCE PUSHUP

Start with your hands wider than shoulder width. Keep your feet to-gether and your back straight. Lower yourself so your chest nearly touches the floor. Return to the starting position. Repeat. Compared to the standard pushup, this variation works the shoulders and upper back more intensively.

105

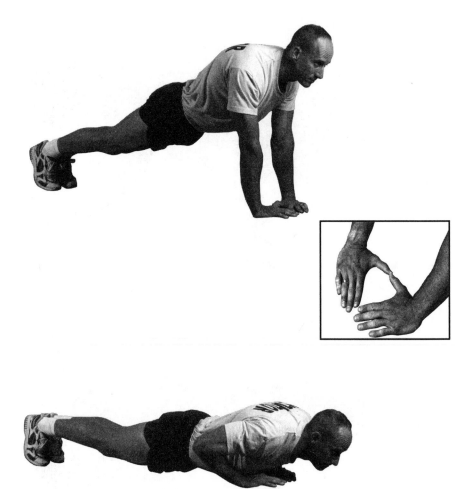

NARROW STANCE PUSHUP

Narrow stance pushups target the triceps in addition to the chest. Key to performing this pushup variation is forming a small diamond with your thumbs and index fingers (see photo detail). Spread your legs a couple of feet apart to enhance stability or, for a real challenge, keep your feet together as shown above. Lower yourself so your chest meets your hands. Return to the starting position.

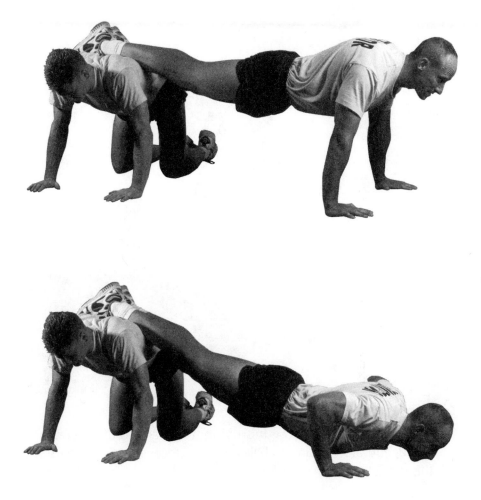

INCLINE PUSHUP

This one requires the assistance of your workout buddy. If you are working out alone, you can use a bench or a stable chair instead. Either way, you're going to have fun cranking these out. Why raise your legs as shown? This way you'll add to the intensity of a standard pushup.

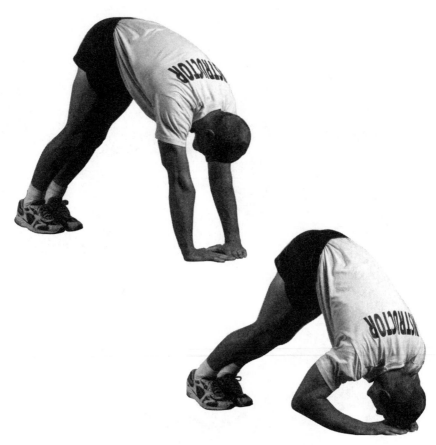

CHINESE PUSHUP

No one is quite sure how this one got its name. But whatever it's called, you are certain to challenge your triceps and shoulders with this difficult pushup variation.

Begin this one from a standing position. Lean over as if to touch your toes, then walk your hands forward until you reach the starting position as shown. Form a diamond with your index fingers and thumbs, just like the narrow stance pushup. Now lower yourself so your forehead meets your hands. Return to the starting position. Congratulations, you've successfully performed one Chinese pushup.

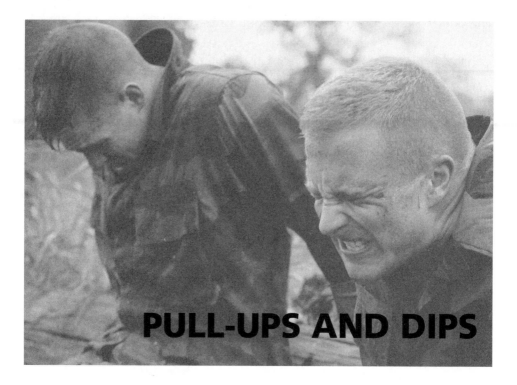

PULL-UPS AND DIPS

H ere are a few tips to keep in mind when performing pull-ups:

- Keep your back arched.
- Think of your arms as a set of hooks—try not to bring your biceps into play too much.
- Isolate your back. Pull-ups are a back exercise, though your arms will inevitably get a solid workout, too.
- Don't forget to stretch beforehand.

Here are three ways to increase the number of pull-ups and pull-up variations you can achieve:

First, use a lat pull-down machine, adding weight up to 10 or 25 pounds more than your body weight. Do five solid pull-downs. Then reduce the weight to 10 or 25 pounds below your body weight and go for eight or nine pull-downs. With this technique you're getting

109

accustomed to doing more of the pull-up movement, plus you're adding resistance. It will make lifting your own body weight easier when doing actual pull-ups.

A second way to increase your ability to perform proper Air Force pull-ups (no bicycling or kicking your legs to get up and over the bar) is to work out with a buddy. Your buddy can actually assist you by pushing upward on your hips or on your lower back, just enough to help you squeeze out a couple more on the pull-up bar.

A third way is to do negatives. A negative is simply a pull-up in reverse. Start from the "up" position. You can get there any way you want. (Some people use a chair.) Now that you are in the "up" position, slowly lower yourself to the down position. Repeat as needed.

Whatever the method, there is no better way to improve at pull-ups than doing pull-ups! Good luck.

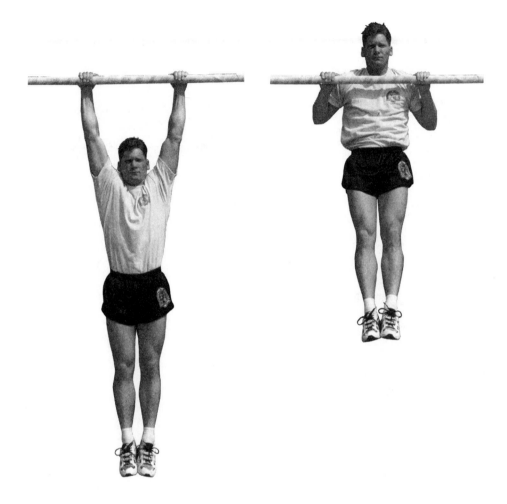

STANDARD PULL-UP

Grab the pull-up bar with your arms spread a little wider than your shoulders. Keep your thumb and fingers on the same side of the bar. From a dead-hang, thinking of the arms as hooks, work your back, not your arms. Keep your back arched. Look up. Pull yourself up over the bar and lower yourself in a controlled fashion. Concentrate on utilizing proper technique for all of the pull-up variations.

111

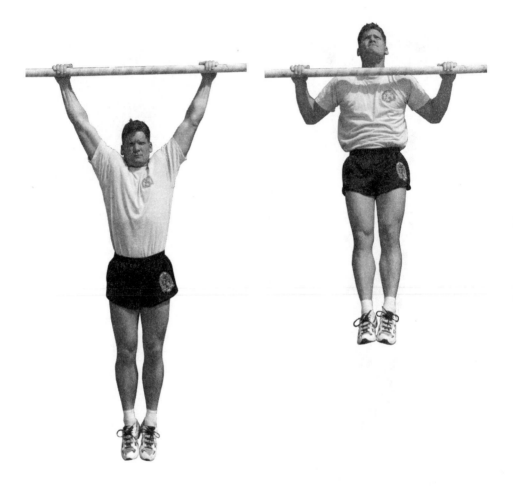

WIDE GRIP PULL-UP

Wide grip pull-ups are definitely challenging. Set your arms as wide as possible—but not so you're uncomfortable. Pull yourself up and lower yourself down. Your back and deltoids will get a great workout.

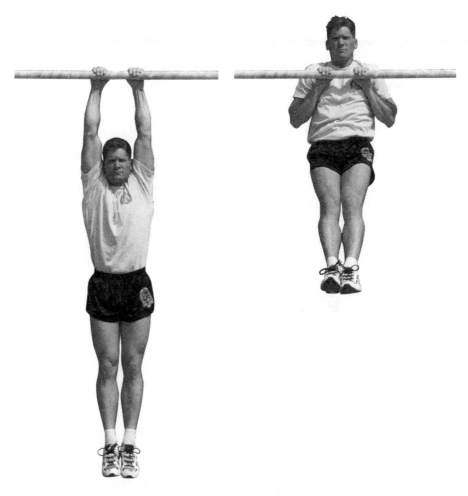

NARROW GRIP PULL-UP

Grab the pull-up bar palms facing out, your hands a couple of inches apart. Use the same technique as in the regular grip pull-up. Back arched. Hands like hooks. Do them right. Notice in the photo the true dead-hang. There is absolutely no leg motion whatsoever. If you are having trouble keeping your legs still, or if you are on the tall side, you might want to bend your knees a bit and cross your legs at the ankles. This will increase your stability and will reduce the tendency to bicycle your legs to gain momentum.

113

Advanced Tip:
Just for the love of a challenge, INDOC instructors like to have their students perform standard pull-ups behind the neck. Behind the neck? Yes. Both the regular and wide pull-ups can be done this way. Just be careful and wait until you can perform the basic pull-ups with ease before trying this advanced variation.

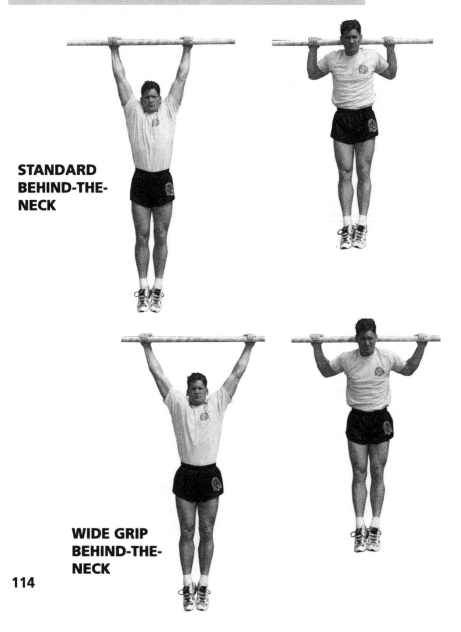

STANDARD BEHIND-THE-NECK

WIDE GRIP BEHIND-THE-NECK

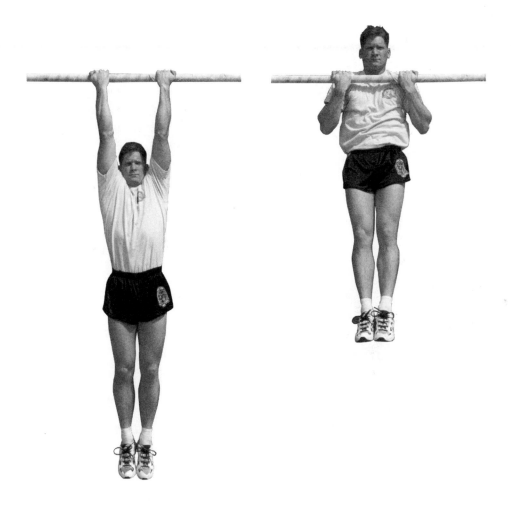

STANDARD CHIN-UP

To perform a proper chin-up, reverse your grip so your palms are facing toward you (again keeping fingers and thumbs on the same side of the bar). Set your hands a few inches apart and perform the exercise. You will find this pull-up variation uses more biceps strength than the others.

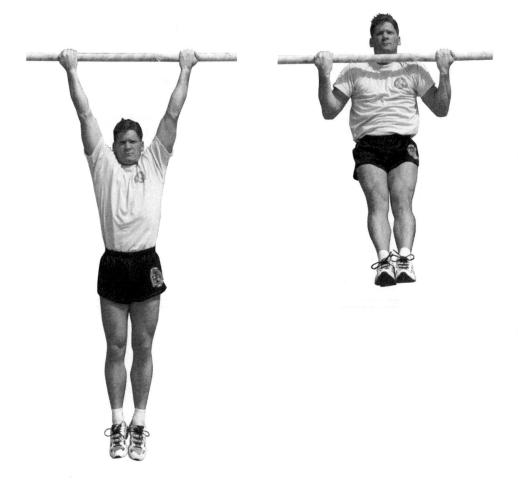

WIDE GRIP CHIN-UP

A variation of the standard chin-up. Spread your arms wider this time. Again, this variation provides a great workout for your back and deltoids.

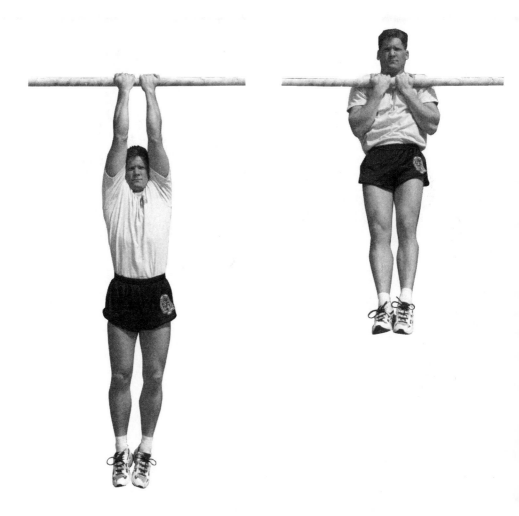

NARROW GRIP CHIN-UP

Another variation. Move those hands close together.

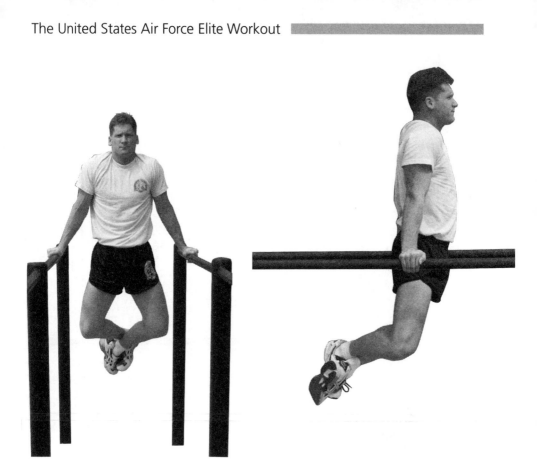

DIPS

A staple in the USAF fitness arsenal! While performing dips keep in mind that proper form is essential. Keep your back straight and slightly arched, and make sure to keep your elbows pointed in. Lower yourself in a controlled manner until your elbows are at a 90° angle. Come up in a smooth motion.

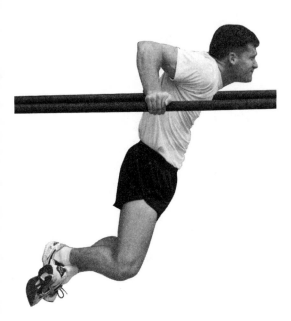
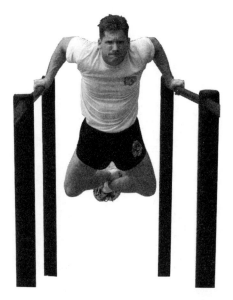

Advanced Tip:
If you want to work your chest more, look down and it will put more stress on your chest. If you want to work your triceps more, look up and you'll be working your triceps more.

ABS AND MIDSECTION

INDOC instruction like to work the abs and midsection. If you practice, with proper form and technique, you'll minimize the pain! Remember, keep your back arched, and let your stomach muscles do the work, not your neck. This section includes variations of ab exercises to work all the muscles in your midsection.

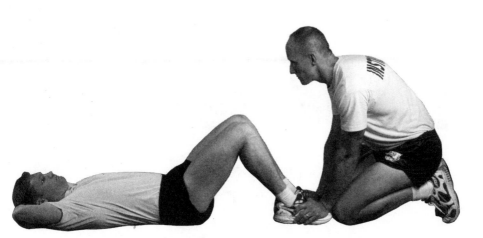

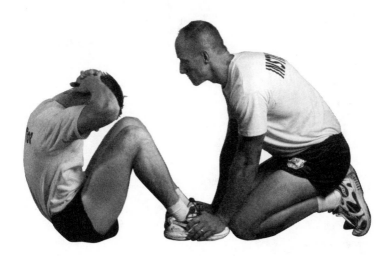

STANDARD SITUP

Another PAST requirement. Learn to do them right: With your work-out buddy holding down your ankles, start with knees bent, at a comfortable angle, hands clasped behind the head, as shown. Now sit up, so your forehead almost touches your knees. Return to the start and repeat.

123

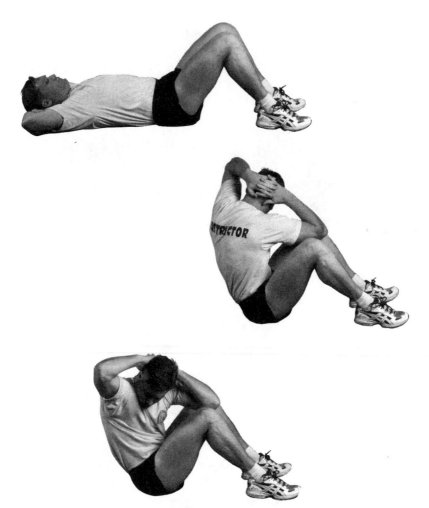

ROCKY SITUP

Yo Adrian! This one is inspired by Sly himself, Sly Stallone that is. Start like you are going to do a regular situp, only this time as you come up, twist your torso so your right elbow touches your left knee, then twist to touch your left elbow to your right knee. When you are in the "up and twisting" position, say "Yo Adrian." Really. Then return to the starting position and repeat. This is all performed in one smooth and fluid motion.

No kidding. This is exactly how the PJ and CCT candidates do it. So the count is, "Yo Adrian, ONE," "Yo Adrian, TWO," etc.

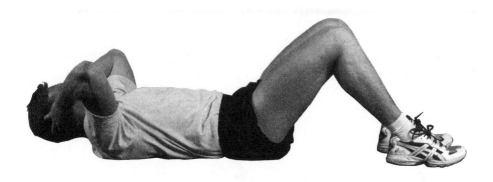

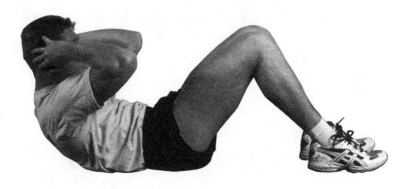

LEG-DOWN CRUNCH

Start with your hands behind your head as shown, knees bent, and using your abs, lift yourself to the crunch position. Do it slowly and with a controlled motion to get the most out of this crunch. Avoid pulling your head up with your hands! This is a sure way to strain your neck and cause injury.

125

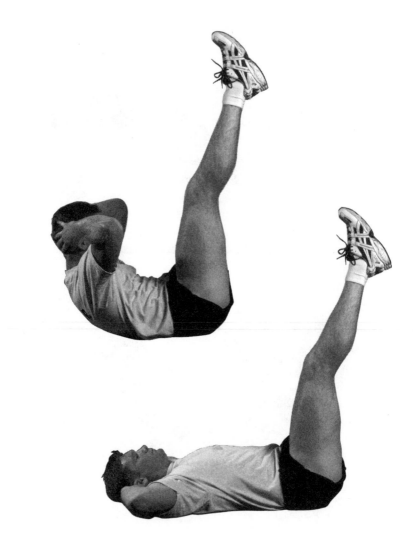

LEG-UP CRUNCH

The legs-up crunch is another variation. Keeping your legs in the air by extending your legs vertically, as shown, creating a 90° angle at the hips, adds to the intensity of the crunch. Do these slowly and hold the crunch position for a two count if you desire an even greater challenge.

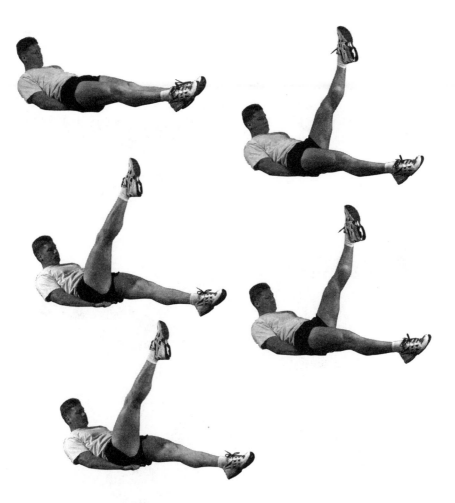

FLUTTER KICKS

Flutter kicks are a great way to strengthen your hip flexors—muscles used consistently during swimming. Flutter Kicks are a requirement of the PAST.

To begin, take your hands and form a sort of "cradle" for your body (see photo). This arm position encourages the back to stay rounded—again to reduce the risk of injury or strain. With your back rounded on the ground, lift your feet about six inches off the ground. Start kicking. Keep your range of motion between six inches to 36 inches maximum. This is a four-count exercise. One, two, three, ONE. One, two, three, TWO. One, two, three, THREE, etc.

127

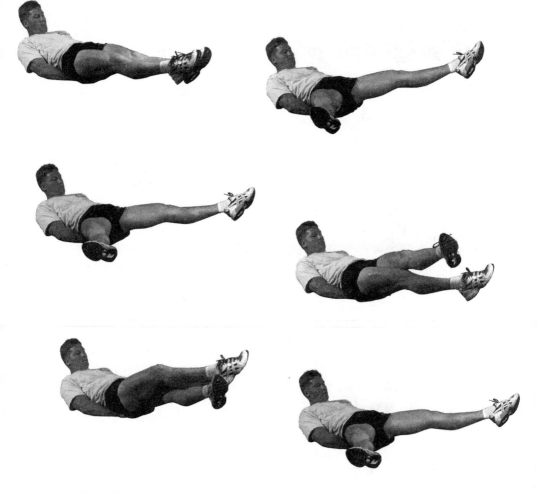

SCISSOR KICKS

Scissor kicks are another great way to strengthen your midsection. Lie on your back, cradling your torso with your arms as you did with flutter kicks. Extend your legs out fully and keep your heels six inches off the floor. Open and close your legs as shown in the photo above. As you bring your legs together, cross your left leg over your right leg. Now open your legs again. Bring them together, this time crossing the right leg over the left as shown. Keep your heels off the floor at all times and perform this exercise uninterrupted as one smooth continuous series of actions.

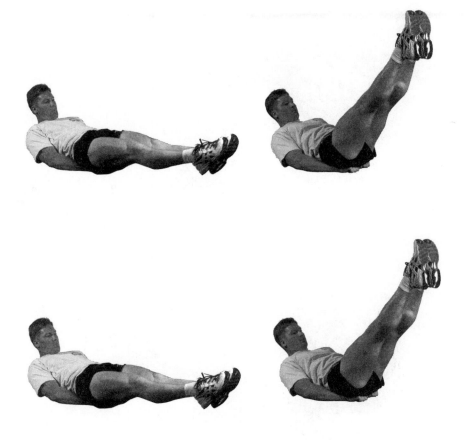

LEG RAISES

Leg raises are a lower abdominal exercise. Start with the same position as the flutter kick with your feet about six inches off the ground. Don't lock your legs out straight; keep them a little flexed. Concentrate on using your lower abs and lift your legs from six inches up to 30 inches, maximum. Lower to the starting position and repeat.

129

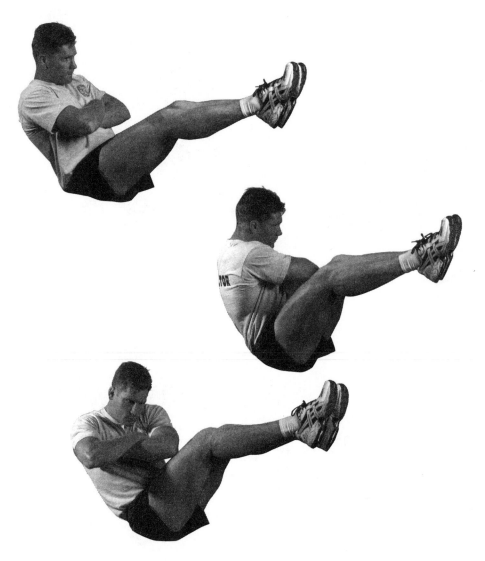

MAD RUSSIANS

What else do you do during those long cold Russian winters? Physical training! This one exercise is certainly worth adding to your fitness training routine. Start with your buttocks on the floor, arms folded across your chest, and your legs held about 12"–16" off the deck. Now twist your torso so your right elbow touches your left knee, then twist so your left elbow touches your right knee. All the while, keep those feet in the air. And have fun!

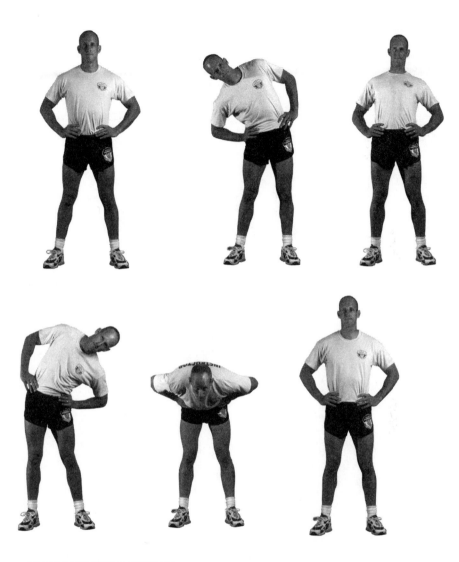

TRUNK TWISTERS

Trunk twisters are a great warm-up exercise, but also help stretch and strengthen the abdominals and lats. Start standing with your feet shoulder width apart and your hands on your hips. This is a rotation exercise, with your hips as the center point. Start by rotating to the right, continue to the back, to the left, and then to the front. Reverse direction after a few cycles to the right. As with all exercises that involve the lower back and spine, remember to be gentle!

131

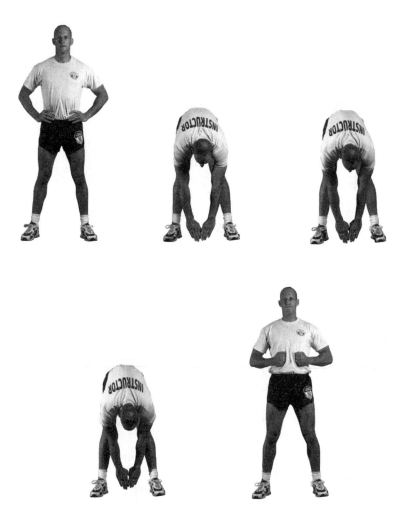

CHERRY PICKERS

Pick those cherries off the ground and put them in your pockets! Well, sort of. Here we are warming up and toning lower back, abs, and hamstrings. Start with your legs spread shoulder width apart and your hands on your hips. On the count of ONE, bend at the waist and reach down to touch the floor ahead of your toes. On TWO, reach to touch the floor at the middle of your feet. On THREE reach a bit further back and try to touch the floor by your heels. On FOUR, rise to the starting position and, with your fists, strike your belly. Hooyah! Make that tummy red! (Your instructors like to see you're trying hard.)

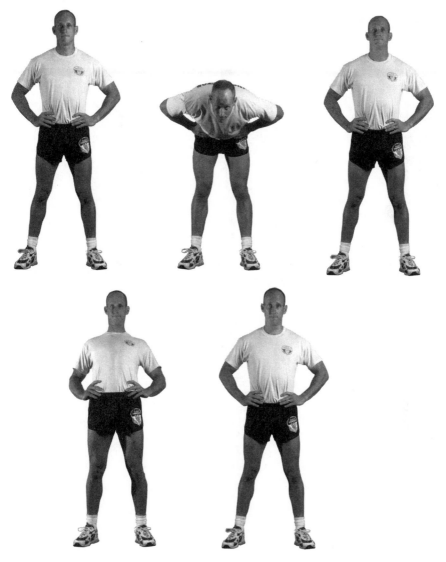

FORE & AFTS

Fore and Afts are simple. Hands on your hips, feet about shoulder width apart. Bend to the front. One. Return to the starting position. Two. Bend to the rear. Three. Return. Four.

As in all exercises, keep an even tempo as you count the repetitions. One, two, three, ONE. One, two, three, TWO. One, two, three, THREE. And so on. It keeps your mind clear so you can remember how many you've done. Or how many more you have to do!

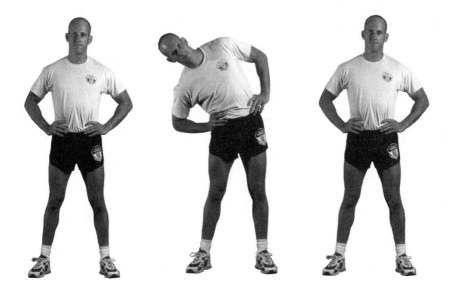

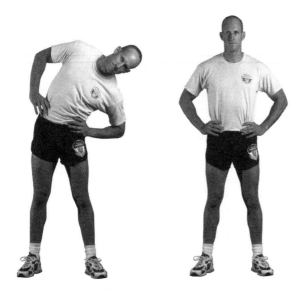

SIDE BENDERS

Another four-count warm-up and strengthening exercise, start your side benders with your feet about shoulder width apart and hands on your hips. On ONE, bend to the right (stretching your left lats). On TWO, return to the starting position. On THREE, bend to your left (stretching your right lats). On FOUR return to start. Repeat.

JUST FOR FUN: EXTRA PT EXERCISES

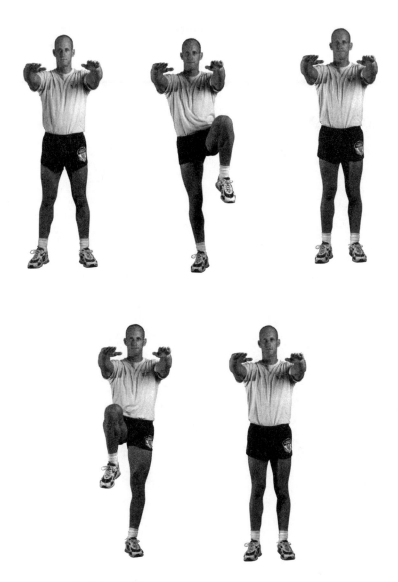

STEAM ENGINES

Combining high kicks with ab crunches, Steam Engines are a great warm-up and a great exercise. Performed as a continuous motion, alternate lifting your right knee and left knee as if to meet your outstretched hands. A you come up, squeeze your abdominal muscles to maximize the overall benefit of the motion. You can also do this as a field drill, moving forward with each kick upward.

137

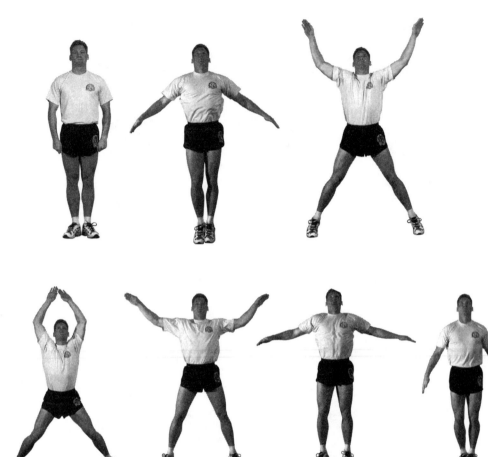

JUMPING JACKS

Begin with your feet together and your arms by your sides. As you jump up, your feet should come apart and your hands should go over your head. Jump again and as you land, bring your feet back together. Jumping Jacks are a great total body warm-up and cardio exercise.

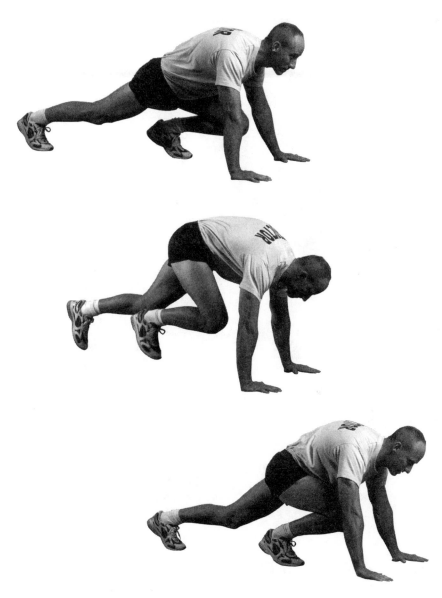

MOUNTAIN CLIMBERS

You might feel like you've climbed Mount Everest once you're done with these! With your hands on the floor, and your arms holding your head high, alternate thrusting your left and right leg behind you as shown. Add a bit of a bounce as you do them, and keep the motion smooth and continuous.

139

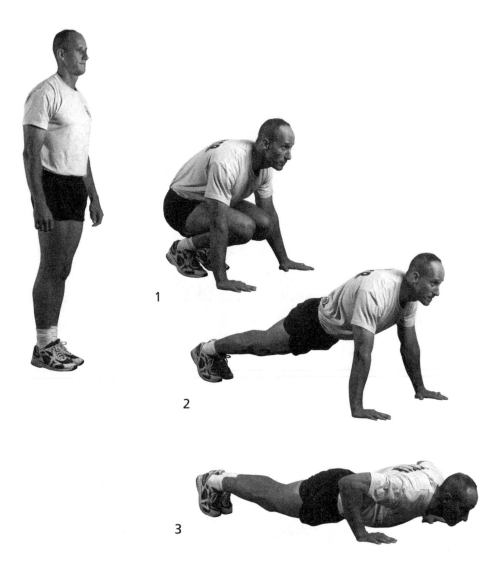

1

2

3

EIGHT-COUNT BODY BUILDERS

The Eight-Count Body Builder is a PT classic. It really is a unique exercise combining a variety of moves and muscles, and the result is a powerful PT exercise that works the upper body, lower body, and cardiorespiratory system.

Begin in a standing position, move to a squat position with your arms slightly more than shoulder width apart and count "ONE." Thrust your legs straight back, count "TWO." Keeping your back

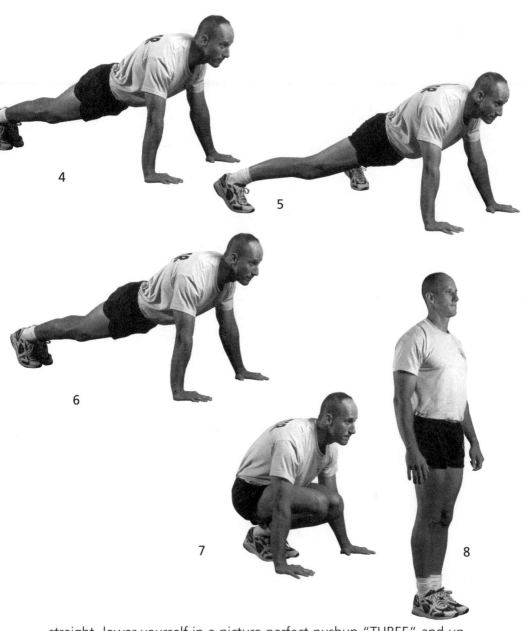

straight, lower yourself in a picture perfect pushup "THREE" and up "FOUR." Kick your legs apart like a scissor "FIVE" then kick them back together "SIX." Pull your legs back in a reverse thrust motion "SEVEN." And stand "EIGHT." You've just completed one Eight-Count Body Builder.

141

THE PJ/CCT INDOC SCHOOL
OBSTACLE COURSE

Candidate Course trainees really get to see what they're made of when it comes time for the obstacle course. This intensive 21-obstacle course spans over one mile and guarantees to challenge upper and lower body strength, agility, balance, and running endurance.

Don't be fooled, this obstacle course is vastly different from that found on the jogging trail of your local park. Here, we are talking about 29-foot walls, barbed wire trenches, and unstable logs—all of which pose a risk to the participant's safety. The 21 obstacles are built on a path approximately one mile long and ends with a tenth of a mile sprint to the finish.

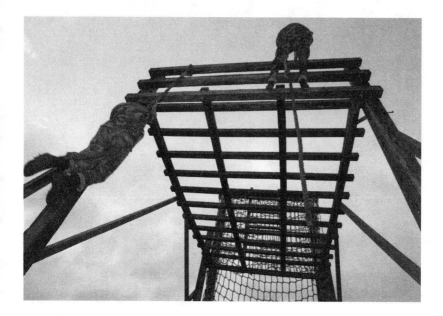

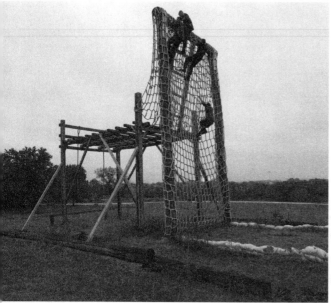

You can see where the name comes from!

THE TOUGH ONE

The first obstacle carries a high safety risk. Team members must climb this 29-foot netting, go over the top log, descend the ladder, and cross the log platform. At the end of the platform, there is a log to go over and then a rope to get to the ground. The team member must vault or belly roll over the final log. There are plenty of opportunities to lose grip on the netting or fall between the logs of the platform so caution is necessary!

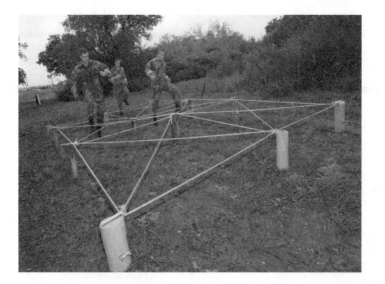

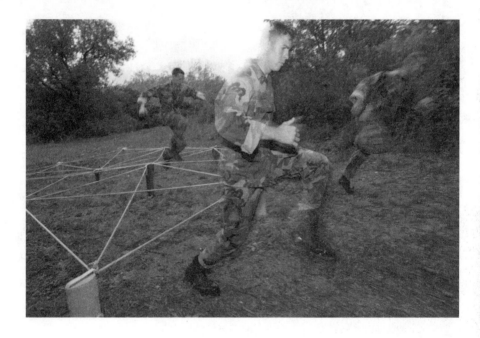

TANGLE FOOT

That's exactly what these ropes are designed to do to you—if you're not agile! Select a lane and move across by stepping into each section of the lane without tripping and falling to the ground. Step high!

145

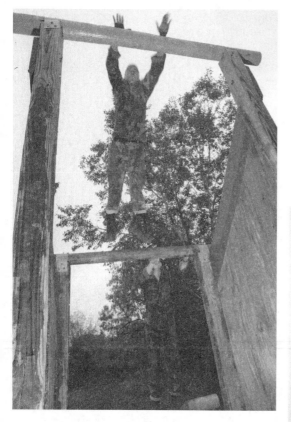

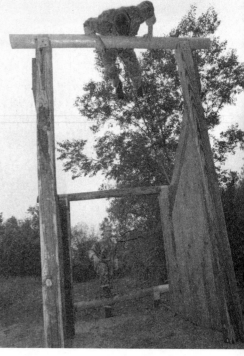

THE DIRTY NAME

One look at this obstacle and it's easy to understand how it got its name. The proper way to negotiate the Dirty Name is to mount the lower log and reach higher logs in succession by jumping to them. Insufficient height when jumping from the second tier to the top log could mean a painful fall forward or backward.

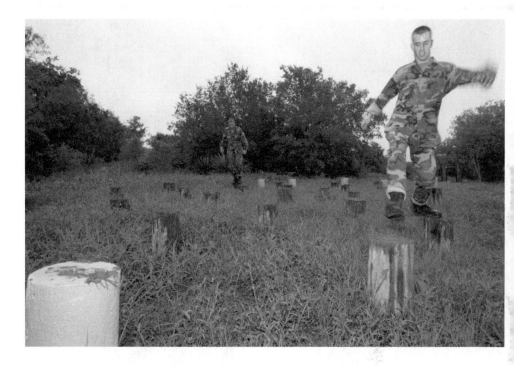

ISLAND HOPPER

Just like jumping from rock to rock across a brook, the goal is to jump from log to log without falling in between. Balance plays a key role in keeping you on your feet.

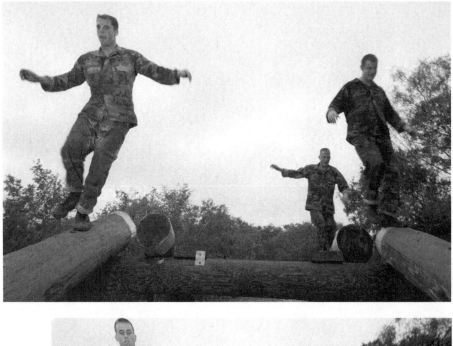

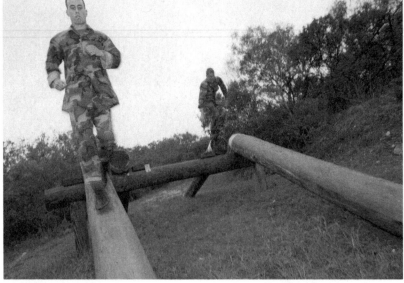

EASY BALANCER

Easy??—a rather misleading name. You must walk or run up one inclined log and down another on the opposite side without falling to the ground. Not only are the logs on a steep incline, accomplishing this successfully means that your hands never touch the logs.

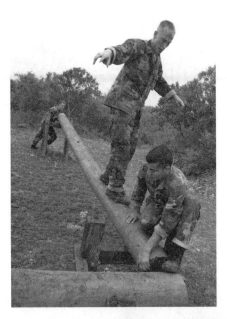

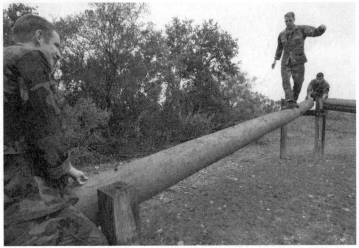

BALANCING LOGS

Adept on the balance beam? If so, you're in luck, except that these are not stationary and are far off the ground. The goal here is to walk or run along the three logs without falling off or ever touching the logs with hands.

THE BELLY BUSTER

Whether it's by vaulting, jumping or climbing, you must get over this unstationary horizontal log without getting any help from the support braces.

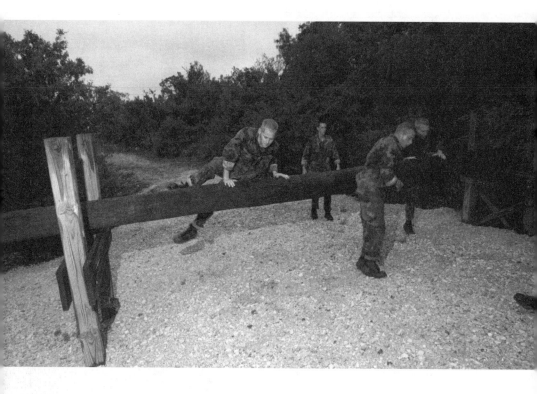

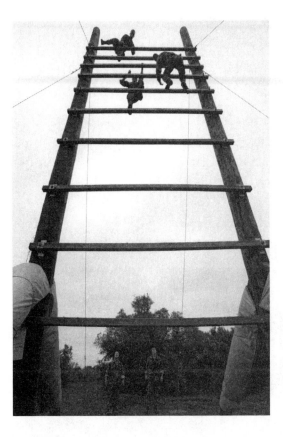

CONFIDENCE CLIMB

The goal here is to climb the vertical ladder, go over the top, and descend down the other side. The distance from bottom to top is about 30 feet so a careful grip is critical to prevent serious injury from a fall. Fear of heights? Not in the Air Force!

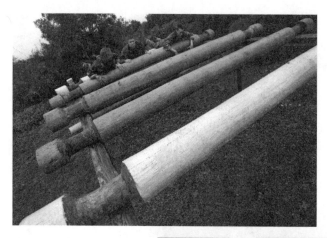

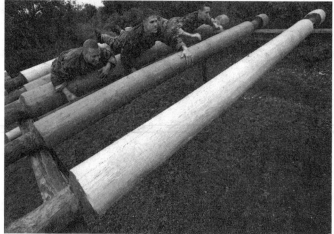

BELLY ROBBER

Face forward, crawl over all the horizontal logs to the end. On your belly. That's right your belly. One try and you'll see how this obstacle got its name.

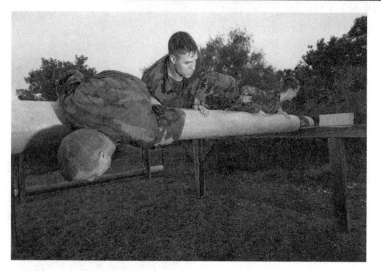

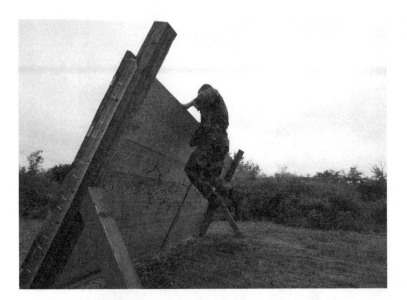

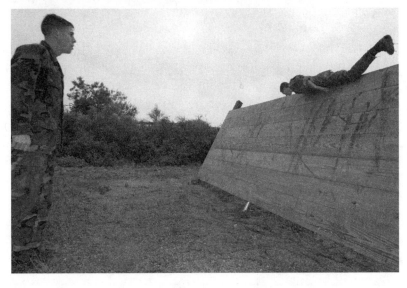

INCLINING WALL

Gaining adequate height to jump up and grasp the top from the underside of the wall is key to pulling your body up and over it. Seeking help from the support braces is not an option.

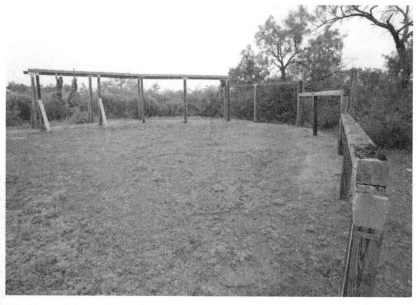

THE TARZAN

You must use Tarzan's balance and skill to get through this one. Begin by mounting the lower log and walking or running the length of it and each successive higher log until you've reached the horizontal ladder without falling to the ground. Then cross the underside of the ladder, hand-over-hand.

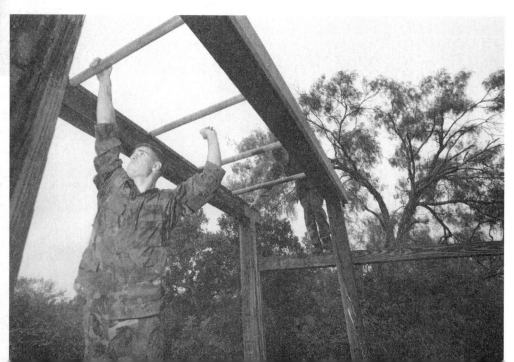

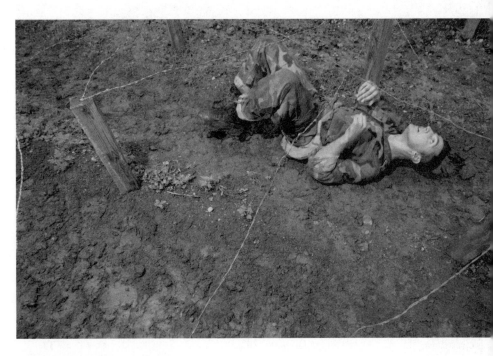

THE TRENCH CRAWL

Warning: lay low! Select a trench and crawl through from start to finish. If you don't stay sufficiently low to the ground, the barbed wire will claw you up.

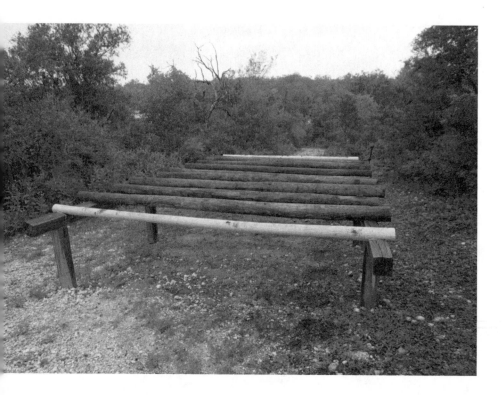

THE HIGH STEPOVER

Cross very carefully—groin injury potential is high. The key is stepping high over each log, one at a time, touching the ground with at least one foot between each row of logs. Yes, hands can and should be used for support.

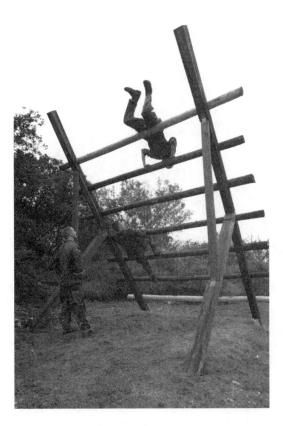

REVERSE CLIMB

Not only is it a ladder, but a ladder on a steep incline. Completion entails climbing the inclined ladder from the underside, going over the top rung, and descending the opposite side head first to the ground. Balance and grip are critical to avoiding a fall and resulting injury.

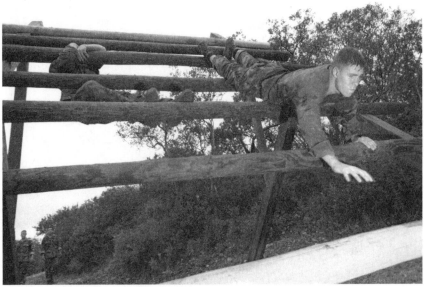

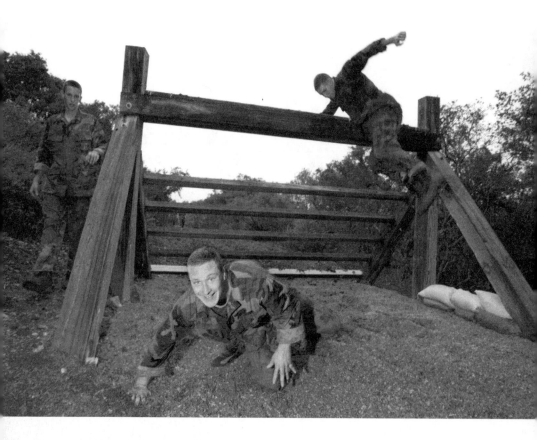

JUMP AND LAND

Another inclined ladder but this time you don't climb down—you jump off, landing on two feet. Bend your knees when you land.

THE WALK ACROSS

Whatever sense of balance you have . . . now's the time to use it! Walk or run along the three beams without falling.

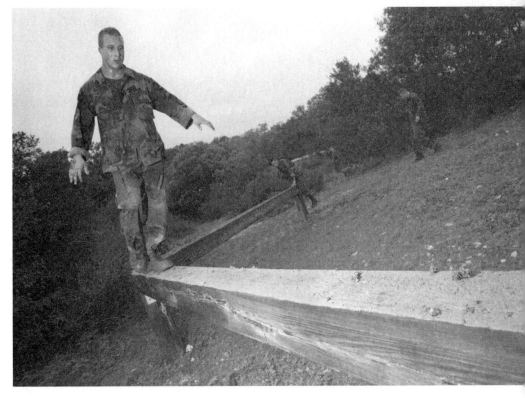

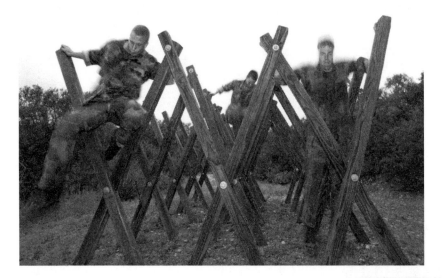

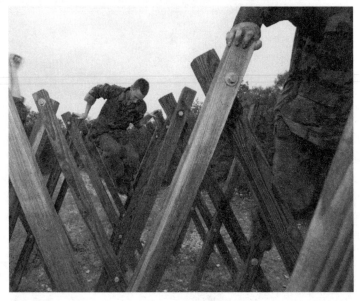

THE TOUGH NUT

Call them modified hurdles, these wooden X's form rows that you must move through by going over every X. Once a row is selected, there is no changing to another. Fortunately, use of hands is allowed to assist in stepping over the X's, but at least one foot must touch the ground between each row.

BELLY CRAWL

Choose a lane, drop to your stomach, and crawl forward under the barbed wire. Press your body to the ground as much as you can! Otherwise you'll find you've shredded your nice shirt on the fiercely jagged wire.

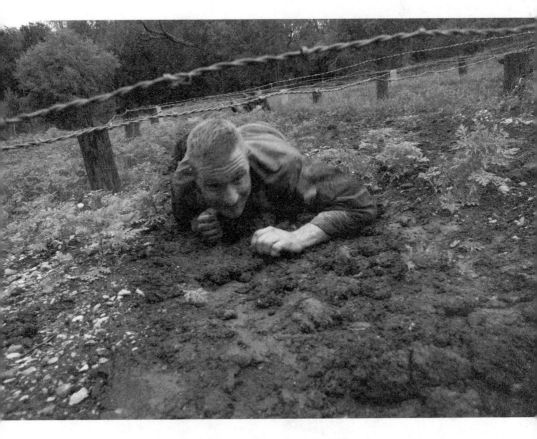

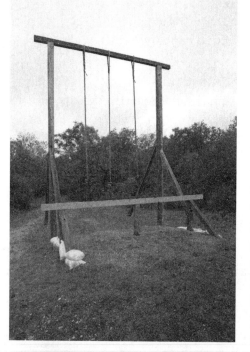

SWING, STOP AND JUMP

The goal here is very precise—grasp a rope with both hands, swing the body forward, and land with both feet on top of the horizontal beam, then jump to the ground. Timing is everything! Too easily a swing can result in a badly bruised chin because you'll hit the log short. Too much swing and you'll overshoot, hitting your head square on the beam.

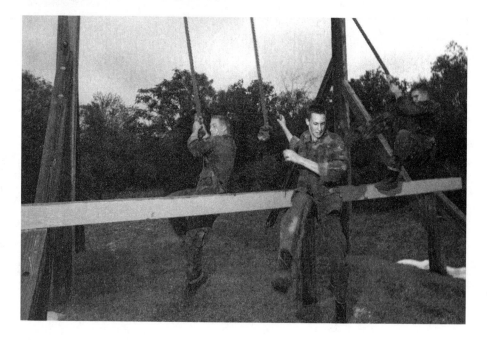

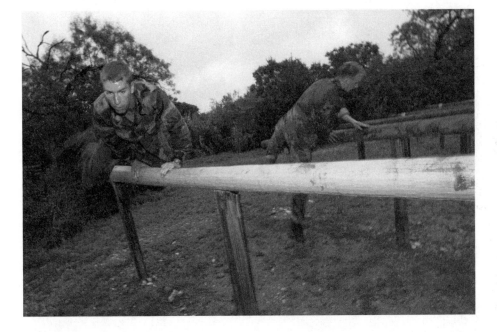

SIX VAULTS
Move swiftly across this series of logs by vaulting or rolling over belly-side. Sufficient height is the sure way to avoid any groin injuries.

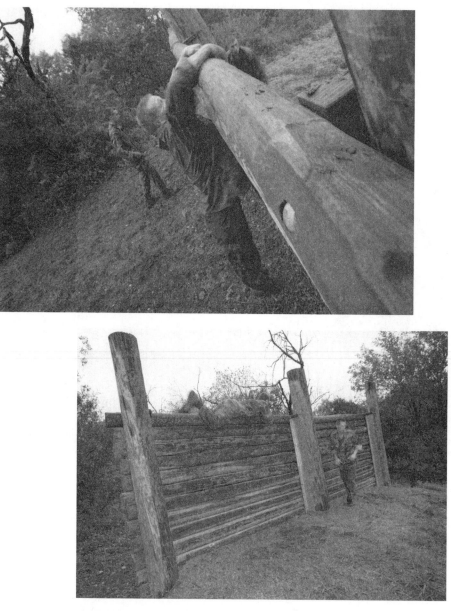

THE VERTICAL WALL

Last, but not least, finish up the obstacles by climbing the vertical wall, going over the top, sliding or jumping to the ground.

The very last part of the course is a sprint, the completion of which indicates the end! Hoo-yah!

10 WEEK PHYSICAL FITNESS SCHEDULE

H ere's an actual start-to-finish schedule of fitness training activities encountered by students at the PJ/CCT Candidate Course, Lackland Air Force Base, Texas. Events listed occur throughout the day in the order shown. This schedule is provided to give you insight into the amount of physical training that occurs during this time. You can also adapt this schedule to provide a foundation for a workout program suitable for your own personal fitness goals.

Note: All swims, with the exception of the PAST, are performed with the student wearing fins.

WEEK 1

Monday
No physical activity scheduled

Tuesday
Swim Evaluation
Run Evaluation
Calisthenics Evaluation

Wednesday
Introduction to Water Confidence Training
Introduction to Swim Training

Thursday
Introduction to Run Training and Stretching
Introduction to Calisthenics
Lifesaving

Friday
Run
Water Confidence Training
Swim Training

WEEK 2

Monday
Run
Calisthenics
Swim Training (distance)
Water Confidence Training

Tuesday
30-minute Long Slow Distance Run
Circuit Training (1 Rep max A/R)
Water Confidence Training
Swim Training

Wednesday
Motivation Schedule*

Thursday
Motivation Schedule*

Friday
Motivation Schedule*

The Motivation Schedule presents a non-stop barrage of different events designed to test the commitment of the students and their desire to become PJs or CCTs.

WEEK 3

Monday
Run Evaluation
Calisthenics Evaluation
Swim Training Evaluation
Water Confidence Training

Tuesday
35-minute Long Slow Distance Run
Introduction to Rope Climbing
Calisthenics or Weight Training
Water Confidence

Wednesday
3-mile Track Run (21 minutes)
Calisthenics
Swim Training (Boerne Reservoir)

Thursday
Introduction to Grass and Guerrilla Drills
Swim Training (distance)
Water Confidence Training

Friday
Interval Training
Calisthenics
Swim Training (sprints)
Water Confidence Training

WEEK 4

Monday
Run Evaluation
Calisthenics Evaluation
Swim Training Evaluation (distance)
Water Confidence Training

Tuesday
45-minute Long Slow Distance Run
Calisthenics or Weight Circuit Training

Wednesday
4-mile Run (28 minutes)
Swim Training (2000 m distance)
Water Confidence Training

Thursday
Introduction to the Obstacle Course
Swim Training (distance)
Water Confidence Training

Friday
Run Interval Training
Calisthenics
Swim Training (sprints)
Water Confidence Training

WEEK 5

Monday
Run Evaluation
Calisthenics Evaluation
Swim Training Evaluation
Water Confidence Training Appraisal

Tuesday
50-minute Long Slow Distance Run
Calisthenics
Water Confidence Training

Wednesday
Swim Training A/R (2500 m)

Thursday
4.5-mile Run (32 minutes)
Guerrilla Drills
Swim Training
Water Confidence Training

Friday
Run Intervals
Calisthenics
Swim Training (sprints)
Water Confidence Training

WEEK 6

Monday
Run Evaluation
Calisthenics Evaluation
Swim Training Evaluation
Water Confidence Training
Evaluation

Tuesday
55-minute Long Slow Distance Run
Calisthenics or Weight Circuit Training
Water Confidence Training

Wednesday
5-mile Run (35 minutes)
Calisthenics

Thursday
Grass/Guerilla Drills
Swim Training (3000 m distance)
Water Confidence Training

Friday
Run Intervals
Calisthenics
Swim Training (sprints)
Water Confidence Training

WEEK 7

Monday
Run Evaluation
Calisthenics Evaluation
Swim Training Evaluation
Water Confidence Training
Evaluation

Tuesday
60-minute Long Slow Distance Run
Calisthenics or Weight Circuit
Training
Water Confidence Training

Wednesday
5.5-mile Run (39 minutes)
Calisthenics

Thursday
Obstacle Course
Swim Training (3500 m)
Water Confidence Training

Friday
Run Intervals
Calisthenics
Swim Training
Water Confidence Training

WEEK 8

Monday
Run Evaluation
Calisthenics Evaluation
Swim Training Evaluation
Water Confidence Training
Evaluation

Tuesday
Obstacle Course
Calisthenics or Circuit Training
Water Confidence or Swim Training

Wednesday
6-mile Run (42 minutes, 30 seconds)
Calisthenics
Water Confidence Training

Thursday
Calisthenics/Circuit Training
Swim Training (4000 m)
Water Confidence Training

Friday
Run Intervals
Water Confidence Training

WEEK 9

Monday
Run Final Evaluation
Calisthenics Final Evaluation
Swim Training Final Evaluation
Water Confidence Training Final
Evaluation

Tuesday
No physical activity scheduled

Wednesday
No physical activity scheduled

Thursday
No physical activity scheduled

Friday
Re-training for:
>   Runs
>   Calisthenics
>   Swimming
>   Water Confidence

WEEK 10

Monday
Re-evaluation for:
>   Runs
>   Calisthenics
>   Swimming
>   Water Confidence

Tuesday
No physical activity scheduled.

Wednesday
No physical activity scheduled.

Thursday
Graduation Run

Friday
Graduation Day!

MEET YOUR INSTRUCTORS

SSGT Tony Alexandar

Staff Sergeant (SSGT) Alexandar began his military career not in the Air Force, but in the Marine Corps. SSGT Alexandar spent six years as a member of the Marine Corps elite Reconnaissance Teams (RE-CON). In 1990, he joined the Air Force to become a Pararescueman. During his career in the Air Force, SSGT Alexandar has been assigned to the 1550th TTW in Albuquerque, New Mexico, the 39th Air Rescue Squadron in Misawa, Japan, and the 33rd Rescue Squadron in Okinawa, Japan.

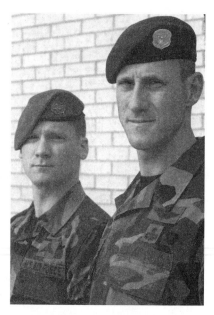

Currently, SSGT Alexandar is an instructor at the PJ/CCT Indoctrination School (INDOC) at Lackland AFB, Texas. He has served in Operation Provide Comfort (Turkey) and Operation Southern Watch (Kuwait) in support of the no fly zones. He has also served in Korea, Malaysia, and Thailand. In his spare time, SSGT Alexandar is an avid mountain biker, rock climber, and skier.

SSGT Alexandar's military training is extensive. Highlights include: US Army Military Freefall Parachutist Course, SOLO Wilderness EMT Course, US Army Special Forces Combat Diver, Aerial Gunnery/Mission Qualification Course, US Army Master Fitness Course, and Airman Leadership School.

SSGT Bill White

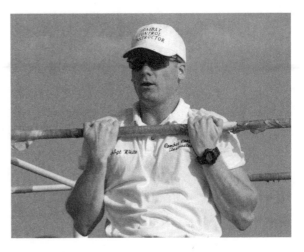

Staff Sergeant White has been a Combat Controller for almost 10 years. Since 1990, he has participated in a wide array of operational activities, including numerous joint special operations exercises and real-world contingencies. He has served with the 1721st Combat Control Squadron, Pope AFB, North Carolina, and the 24th Special Tactics Squadron, also stationed at Pope AFB.

At present, SSGT White is a PJ/CCT INDOC Course Instructor at Lackland Air Force Base, Texas. He is a Military Freefall Jumpmaster, Dive Supervisor, and a certified personal trainer. In his spare time, Bill is an avid triathlete and rock climber.

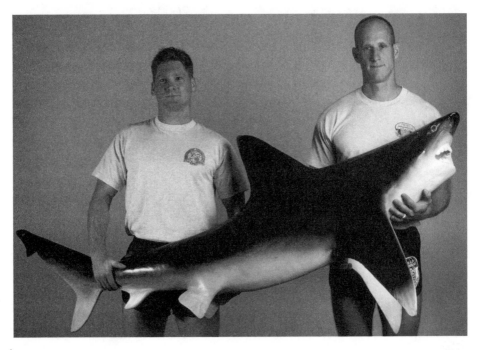

Candidate Course Standards

These are the actual standards by which the INDOC students are tested weekly. Note the progression of both distance and time for the run and swim evaluations.

	Run (miles/minutes)	Swim (meters/minutes)
Day 1	1.5 / 10:30	1000 / 26:00
Week 1	2.0 / 14:00	1000 / 20:00 (all subsequent weeks w/fins)
Week 2	3.0 / 21:00	1500 / 30:00
Week 3	3.0 / 21:00	1500 / 30:00
Week 4	4.0 / 28:00	2000 / 40:00
Week 5	4.5 / 32:00	2500 / 50:00
Week 6	5.0 / 35:30	3000 / 60:00
Week 7	5.5 / 39:00	3500 / 70:00
Week 8	6.0 / 42:30	4000 / 80:00

	Pull-Ups	Chin-Up	Situps	Pushups	Flutter Kicks
Day 1	7	8	50	50	50
Week 1	7	8	50	50	50
Week 2	8	9	55	50	60
Week 3	8	9	55	55	60
Week 4	9	10	60	55	70
Week 5	10	11	65	60	70
Week 6	11	12	70	60	80
Week 7	12	13	70	65	80
Week 8	13	14	75	70	85

Repetition Sets

Just that—repetitions. And plenty of them! Remember to stretch before and after your workout!

		Week 1	Week 2	Week 3	Week 5+
Warm Ups	**Sets**	**1**	**3**	**3**	**4**
Trunk Twister		5 reps	10 reps	10 reps	12 reps
Cherry Picker		5	10	10	10
Neck Rotations		5	10	10	10
Fore and Afts		5	10	10	10
Side Benders		5	10	10	10
Steam Engines		5	10	10	15
Jumping Jacks		10	20	25	30
Mountain Climbers		10	10	15	20
8-Count Body Builders		5	10	15	17
Back / Biceps	**Sets**	**1**	**3**	**3**	**4**
Behind the Head Pull-Ups					
Standard Grip		3 reps	5 reps	6 reps	8 reps
Wide Grip		3	5	6	8
Narrow Grip		3	5	6	8
Front of the Head Pull-Ups					
Standard Grip		3	5	6	8
Wide Grip		3	5	6	8
Narrow Grip		3	5	6	8

		Week 1	Week 2	Week 3	Week 5+
Chin-Ups					
	Standard	3 reps	5 reps	6 reps	8 reps
	Wide Grip	3	5	6	8
	Narrow Grip	3	5	6	8
Abdominals	**Sets**	**1**	**3**	**3**	**3**
Situps					
	Standard	45 reps	45 reps	50 reps	55 reps
	Rocky	45	45	50	55
Crunches					
	Leg Up	45	45	50	55
	Leg Down	45	45	50	55
	Sequence	10/10/10	20/20/20	25/25/25	30/30/30
Chest / Triceps	**Sets**	**1**	**3**	**4**	**4**
Pushups					
	Standard	35 reps	40 reps	45 reps	50 reps
	Wide Stance	35	40	45	50
	Narrow Stance	35	40	45	50
	Incline	20	25	30	35
	Chinese	8	8	10	10
	Dips	10	10	15	15
Hip Flexors	**Sets**	**1**	**3**	**4**	**4**
	Flutter Kicks	55 reps	60 reps	65 reps	70 reps
	Scissor Kicks	55	60	65	70
	Leg Raises	20	25	30	35

Timed sets

The purpose of timed sets is to guarantee maximum performance by all students, as INDOC trainees possess varying levels of fitness. By performing timed sets, each student does as many as he can in the time allotted. If, on the other hand, repetition sets are performed—for example, everyone does 75 pushups—it would be easy for some students and extremely hard for others.

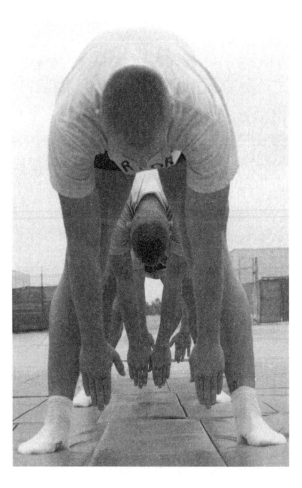

The period of exercise is followed by an equal period of rest. For example, 2 x 50 means two sets of that exercise in 50 seconds of work, followed by 50 seconds of rest.

The specific exercises for timed sets vary from instructor to instructor. The instructor chooses which exercises he will do for those specific body parts.

Here's an example: BACK/BICEPS 2 X 45—This could be accomplished by completing one set of wide grip pull-ups for 45 seconds, then a set of close grip chin-ups for 45 seconds. So if no instructor is present to guide you, select from the exercises found in this book to complete these sets.

Examples of timed sets used in PJ/CCT Training

WEEK	2	3	4	5	6	7	8	9
WARMUP	3x	3x	4x	4x	5x	5x	6x	6x
BACK/	1 x 30	1 x 30	1 x 30	1 x 30	2 x 30	1 x 35	2 x 35	2 x 35
BICEPS	1 x 25	1 x 25	1 x 25	1 x 25	2 x 25	2 x 30	2 x 30	2 x 30
			1 x 20	2 x 20	2 x 20	2 x 20	3 x 20	4 x 20	2 x 25
									2 x 20

ABDOMINALS								
	2 x 30	2 x 35	2 x 40	2 x 45	2 x 45	2 x 50	1 x 60	1 x 60
	2 x 30	2 x 30	2 x 30	2 x 35	2 x 40	2 x 45	2 x 50	2 x 50
				1 x 30	2 x 35	2 x 40	2 x 40	2 x 40
							3 x 30	2 x 30

CHEST/								
TRICEPS	2 x 30	2 x 30	2 x 30	1 x 35	2 x 35	2 x 40	2 x 45	1 x 60
	1 x 15	1 x 25	1 x 25	2 x 30	2 x 30	2 x 30	2 x 40	1 x 45
			1 x 20	2 x 20	2 x 20	2 x 25	4 x 30	1 x 40
							2 x 20	2 x 30
								2 x 25
								1 x 20

HIP								
FLEXORS	2 x 30	2 x 40	2 x 40	2 x 45	2 x 45	2 x 50	1 x 60	1 x 60
	2 x 30	2 x 30	2 x 30	2 x 35	2 x 40	2 x 45	2 x 50	2 x 50
				1 x 30	2 x 35	2 x 40	2 x 40	2 x 40
							3 x 30	2 x 30

179

STUDENT PREPARATION GUIDELINES

The following workouts are taken directly from the Combat Control Pararescue Course Warning Order. These workouts are designed for two categories of people: Category I is for those future Pararescue/Combat Control Candidate Course trainees that have never or have not recently been on a routine PT program. Category II is designed for high school and college athletes that have had a routine PT program. Usually, athletes in sports that require a high level of cardiovascular activity—swimming, running, and wrestling, for example—are in Category II.

Whether you intend to be a PJ or CCT, or just want to be as fit as one, the following guidelines will be extremely helpful as you set out on your fitness journey. Remember to warm up before stretching, stretch before and after exercising, and drink plenty of water before, during, and after your workout. If you feel pain, do not exercise through it. Pain is a warning sign that something may be wrong. Stop and consider what the source of the pain is—a strain, a sprain, fatigue—and take appropriate remedial action.

WORKOUT FOR CATEGORY I

The majority of the physical activities you will be required to perform during your ten weeks of training at the Candidate Course will involve a large amount of running. The intense amount of running can lead to overstress injuries of the lower extremities in the trainees who arrive not physically prepared to handle the activities. Swimming, bicycling, and lifting weights will prepare you for some of the activities at the Candidate Course, but only running can prepare your lower extremities for the majority of the activities.

The goal of Category I is to build up to running 16 miles per week. After you have achieved that goal then and only then should you continue on to the Category II goal of 30 miles of running per training week.

Category I is a nine week "build-up" program. Follow the workout as best as you can and you will be amazed at the progress you will make.

Running Schedule I

Week	Miles Per Day	Miles Per Week
Weeks 1/2	2 miles per day, 8:30 pace M / W / F	6 miles
Week 3	No running (high risk of stress fractures)	
Week 4	3 miles per day, M / W / F	9 miles
Weeks 5/6	2 / 3 / 4 / 2 miles, M / Tu / Th / F	11 miles
Weeks 7/8	3 / 4 / 5 / 2 miles, M / Tu / Th / F	14 miles
Week 9	3 / 4 / 5 / 2 miles, M / Tu / Th / F	14 miles

Physical Training Schedule I

Exercise on Monday, Wednesday, and Friday. For best results, alternate exercises. Do a set of pushups, then a set of situps, followed by a set of pull-ups, with no rest. Rest between sets no more than two minutes. If you are unable to complete the pull-up sequence doing standard exercises, do "negatives." Start in the "up" position. Slowly lower yourself in a controlled fashion to the "down" position. Get back in the "up" position in the easiest manner possible and lower yourself again. Repeat as needed.

Exercises	Sets/ Reps	Exercises	Sets/ Reps
Week 1		**Weeks 5 / 6**	
Pushups	4 x 15	Pushups	6 x 25
Situps	4 x 20	Situps	6 x 25
Pull-ups	3 x 3	Pull-ups	2 x 8
Week 2		**Weeks 7 / 8**	
Pushups	5 x 20	Pushups	6 x 30
Situps	5 x 20	Situps	6 x 30
Pull-ups	3 x 3	Pull-ups	2 x 10
Weeks 3 / 4		**Week 9**	
Pushups	5 x 25	Pushups	6 x 30
Situps	5 x 25	Situps	6 x 30
Pull-ups	3 x 4	Pull-ups	3 x 10

Swimming Schedule I

Swim using either the sidestroke or freestyle method without fins four to five days per week. Each week also complete two to four 25 meter underwater swims.

If you do not have access to a swimming pool, ride a bike for twice as long as you would swim. If you do have access to a pool, swim every day available! Four to five days a week and 200 meters per session is your initial training goal. Work on developing your side stroke on both your left and right sides. For speed, try to swim 50 meters in one minute or less.

Week	Time
Weeks 1 / 2	Swim continuously for 15 minutes.
Weeks 3 / 4	Swim continuously for 20 minutes.
Weeks 5 / 6	Swim continuously for 25 minutes.
Weeks 7 / 8	Swim continuously for 30 minutes.
Week 9	Swim continuously for 35 minutes.

WORKOUT FOR CATEGORY II

Category II is a more intense workout designed for those who have been involved with a routine PT schedule or those who have completed the requirements of Category I. *Do not attempt this workout schedule unless you can complete Week 9 of Category I.*

Running Schedule II

Running days are Monday / Tuesday / Thursday / Friday / Saturday.

Week	Miles Per Day	Miles Per Week
Weeks 1/2	3 / 5 / 4 / 5 / 2 miles	19 miles
Week 3/4	4 / 5 / 6 / 4 / 3 miles	22 miles
Week 5	5 / 5 / 6 / 4 / 4 miles	24 miles
Week 6	5 / 6 / 6 / 6 / 4 miles	27 miles
Week 7	6 / 6 / 6 / 6 / 6 miles	30 miles

For training Weeks 8 / 9 and beyond. **It is not necessary to increase the distance runs. Work on the speed of your 6 mile runs. Try to get your time down to 7:15 per mile or lower. If you wish to increase the distance of your runs, do it gradually—no more than one mile per day increase for every week beyond Week 9.**

Physical Training Schedule II

These workouts are designed for muscle endurance. Muscle fatigue will gradually take longer and longer to occur when you perform high repetitions. For best results, alternate exercises each set, in order to rest the muscle group for a short time. Exercise using proper form. See the pages of this book for illustrations and descriptions of the exercises. Exercise Monday, Wednesday, and Friday.

Exercises	Sets/ Reps	Exercises	Sets/ Reps
Weeks 1 / 2		**Week 5**	
Pushups	6 x 30	Pushups	15 x 20
Situps	6 x 35	Situps	15 x 25
Pull-ups	3 x 10	Pull-ups	4 x 12
Dips	3 x 20	Dips	15 x 15
Weeks 3 / 4		**Week 6**	
Pushups	10 x 20	Pushups	20 x 20
Situps	10 x 25	Situps	20 x 25
Pull-ups	4 x 10	Pull-ups	5 x 12
Dips	10 x 15	Dips	20 x 15

A WORD ABOUT PYRAMID WORKOUTS

Your can perform "pyramids" with any exercise. The challenge is to slowly build up to a goal, then work back down to the beginning of the workout. For instance, pull-ups, situps, and dips can be alternated as in the above workouts, but this time choose a number to be your maximum repetition. Simply work your way up and then back down the pyramid.

Exercise	# Repetitions
Pull-ups	1, 2, 3, 4, 5, 4, 3, 2, 1
Pushups	2, 4, 6, 8, 10, 8, 6, 4, 2 perform 2 sets
Sit-ups	3, 6, 9, 12, 15, 12, 9, 6, 3 perform 3 sets
Dips	2, 4, 6, 8, 10, 8, 6, 4, 2 perform 2 sets

Swimming Workout II

Swim as often as you can, ideally four or five days per week. At first, alternate swimming 1000 meters with fins and 1000 meters without fins. This will reduce the initial stress on your foot muscles when starting with fins. Your speed goal should be to swim 50 meters in :45 seconds or less. Remember to add at least three and as many as five underwater swims per week.

Stretch PT

Since Mondays, Wednesdays. and Fridays are devoted to calisthenics, it is important to devote at least 20 minutes on Tuesday, Thursday and Saturday to stretching.

187

NUTRITION

You can't achieve peak fitness without paying attention to what you eat. Strong dietary habits are critical both before entering training and during the training itself. Optimum performance is achieved by proper nutrient intake and is essential to receiving maximum performance output during exercise. Nutrition also promotes vital muscle and tissue growth and repair. The ideal diet provides all the nutrients that the body needs and supplies energy for exercise.

Balancing energy intake and expenditure can be very difficult when activity levels are very high (as PJ and CCT training) and when activity levels are very low, such as during isolation. Typically, body weight remains constant when energy intake equals expenditure.

If Caloric Intake =	And Caloric Output =	The Result Is
3000	3000	No Change in Weight
4000	2000	Weight Gain
2000	3000	Weight Loss

You can upset this "energy balance equation" by increasing or decreasing the number of calories you consume, increasing or decreasing your energy expenditure, or both. One pound of body fat is equal to 3,500 calories. So to lose 1 pound in 1 week, you'd have to, over the course of the week, consume 3,500 fewer calories, increase your activity level, or a combination of the two. To gain 1 pound in the same time, you'd need to consume 3,500 calories more than you expend, decrease your physical activity, or a combination of both.

COMPONENTS OF ENERGY EXPENDITURE

The three major contributors to energy expenditure are:

- Resting energy expenditure (REE)
- Physical activity
- Energy used to digest foods

The first two contributors are most pertinent to our discussion. Resting energy expenditure (REE) is the amount of energy required to maintain life—your breathing, heartbeat, body temperature regulation, and other vital processes (but not physical exertion). You can estimate your REE with the following formulas.

Calculating Resting Energy Expenditure (REE)
11 x body weight in pounds

To calculate your total daily caloric expenditure you need to account for your physical activity in addition to your REE. The amount of energy expended during Marine Corps training varies from day to day. Some days are very strenuous and involve running, swimming, calisthenics, and carrying heavy loads. Some days are spent in the classroom sitting a good portion of the time. Thus, determining your actual energy expenditure during activity is more difficult. But there are ways to estimate. One is to multiply your REE by an "activity factor."

Estimating Total Daily Energy Needs at Various Levels of Activity

Level of General Activity	Activity Factor
Very Light. Seated and standing activities, driving, playing cards	1.3
Light. Walking, carpentry, sailing, ping-pong, pool, or golf	1.6
Moderate. Carrying a load, jogging, light swimming, biking, calisthenics, scuba diving	1.7
Heavy. Walking uphill with a load, rowing, digging, climbing, soccer, basketball, running, obstacle course	2.1
Exceptional. Running/swimming races, biking uphill, carrying very heavy loads, hard rowing	2.4

Here's an example using a 21-year-old male who weighs 175 pounds and whose activity level is moderate:

REE = 175[1] x 11 = 1,925 calories per day

Total Energy Needs = 1,925 x 1.7[2] = 3,273 calories per day

[1] 175 = weight in pounds

[2] 1.7 = "Moderate" Activity Factor

Body Mass Index

The Body Mass Index (BMI) is a measure commonly used to assess body composition and then classify individuals as underweight, overweight, or overfat. The BMI is a ratio: weight/height,[2] with weight measured in kilograms and height in meters.

The reference ranges developed for the United States population as a whole do not always apply to special populations such as the Air Force CCTs and PJs. For that reason, a BMI reference range based on a survey of 800 Navy SEALs was developed. That range can be used for the Air Force. For all SEALs combined, for example, the average BMI was 25 and the average body fat was 13 percent. What is important to remember is that the index is a screening tool. You can use the BMI to assess and keep track of changes in your body composition. If your BMI is high, have your body fat checked. If it's more than 20 percent, you need to take some action to lower your weight. Reference BMI values for you are provided below:

Reference BMI Values

Lean	<20
Typical	20 to 29
Overfat	29 to 32

EATING FOR OPTIMUM HEALTH

Once you know where you stand in terms of your BMI, caloric intake, and caloric expenditures, it's important to carefully consider your diet. The following section explains the way to build a healthful diet. The information comes from the Dietary Guidelines for Americans released in 2000 by the U.S. Department of Agriculture and the U.S. Department of Health and Human Services. Top dietitians and scientists have studied the practicality and reliability of the data. It is tested, supported, and credentialed.

In this section you'll learn about basic nutrition: Your daily nutrient and caloric needs; vitamins, minerals, and more. From there you'll discover the Food Pyramid. It's a simple yet profound way to understand where your calories should come from. Finally, you'll learn how to read a nutrition label and be able to make intelligent, healthy decisions at the supermarket or even at a fast food restaurant.

THE CHALLENGE OF CHOICE

Good nutrition boils down to two elements: choice and portion size. Choice involves the types of foods you eat and how they're prepared. Are you more apt to eat a baked sweet potato or a plate of fries? An apple or apple pie? Even the simplest choices, such as the decision to forego slabs of butter on your pancakes, can save you hundreds of calories that you probably won't even miss in terms of flavor.

As important as *what* you eat is *how much* of each food you eat. There are no good or bad foods (with the exception of trans-fatty acids, which is covered later). Portion control is the key. In the last few years

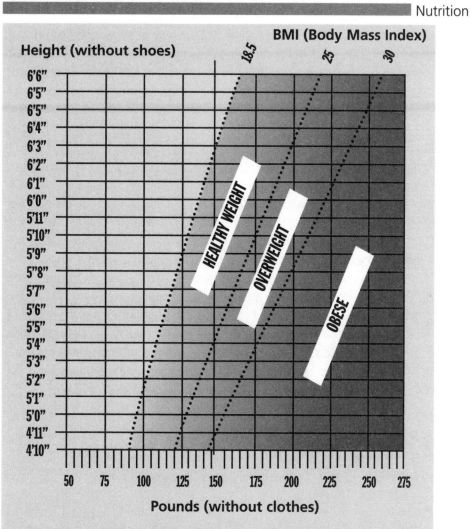

Height (without shoes)

BMI (Body Mass Index)

18.5   25   30

HEALTHY WEIGHT

OVERWEIGHT

OBESE

Pounds (without clothes)

BMI measures weight in relation to height. The BMI ranges shown above are for adults. They are not exact ranges of healthy and unhealthy weights. However, they show that health risk increases at higher levels of overweight and obesity. Even within the healthy BMI range, weight gains can carry health risks for adults.

Directions: Find your weight on the bottom of the graph. Go straight up from that point until you come to the line that matches your height. Then look to find your weight group.

Healthy Weight: BMI from 18.5 up to 25 refers to a healthy weight.
Overweight: BMI from 25 up to 30 refers to overweight.
Obese: BMI 30 or higher refers to obesity. Obese persons are also overweight.

193

portion sizes of virtually all foods—from mega-muffins and "big grab" chips, to cookies, to restaurant entrées—have ballooned. Often, what is sold in single packages really represents two or three servings. In this section you'll also find out how to determine sensible portion sizes based on the Food Guide Pyramid model.

Nutrition Basics

Fad diets come and go, but basic science-backed nutrition advice has remained remarkably consistent. In fact, many reported studies have proven that the best way to lose fat, keep it off, and enjoy a healthful diet is to follow a plan that is rooted not in a new trend, but in the Department of Agriculture's Food Guide Pyramid. While most of us are excited by new trends and fads, the truth is that they don't work in the long term. What does work is a balanced eating and exercising plan that is based on reasonable and attainable goals.

The key to the Food Guide Pyramid is that it provides a wide range of choices so you can eat a variety of tasty foods. Eating a variety of foods ensures that you get all the important nutrients, vitamins, and minerals that your body requires for optimal health. It also means that you won't be bored to death because you can select different foods every day.

DAILY NUTRIENT NEEDS

For a healthy, balanced diet, you need to consume healthful portions of protein, carbohydrates, and fats. Here's the breakdown.

Protein

Protein is made up of chemicals called amino acids. Some types of amino acids, called *nonessential amino acids*, are produced by the body. Nine essential amino acids must come from food you consume. Protein allows the body to build, maintain, and replace body tissue. Muscles, organs, and some hormones are made up primarily of protein. Protein also makes hemoglobin—the part of red blood cells that carries oxygen—and antibodies, the cells that fight off infection and disease.

Good sources of protein include meat, chicken, fish, eggs, cheese, beans, and nuts.

The recommended intake of protein is 50 to 70 grams per day (which should equal 12 to 20 percent of your daily caloric intake).

Carbohydrates

There are two types of carbohydrates: simple and complex. Simple carbohydrates are sugars. They're quickly and easily broken down and digested by the body. Complex carbohydrates, also known as starches, take longer to be digested than simple carbohydrates.

Carbohydrates are the preferred energy source for physical activity. It takes at least 20 hours after demanding exercise to restore muscle energy, provided 600 grams of carbohydrates are consumed each day. During successive days of exhausting training like that of Air Force CCT and PJ training, your energy stores become depleted. A high-carbohydrate diet can help you maintain energy.

Good sources of simple carbohydrates include fruits, such as apples, bananas, grapes, raisins, oranges, and pears. Good sources of complex carbohydrates include bread, cereals, pasta, rice, oatmeal, pretzels, corn, potatoes, sweet potatoes, tomatoes, carrots, cucumbers, lettuce, and peppers.

Normally, the recommended intake of carbohydrates is 350 to 400 grams per day or 55 to 65 percent of your daily intake. During training, however, 600 grams per day or up to 70 percent of your daily caloric intake should be from carbohydrates. Most of that should be from foods high in complex carbohydrates.

Fat

You'll notice that the Food Guide Pyramid allows you to consume 25 to 30 percent of your daily calories from fat. For too long Americans have bought into the myth that fat is evil and that as long as we severely restrict fat intake, we would also control weight. This misconception was based largely on the fact that high-fat foods contain more calories per gram than do other foods. (A single gram of fat has 9 calories; a single gram of carbohydrates and protein has 4 calories.) However, substituting non-fat or low-fat products for fats has not led to success in fat loss. Why? Here are the facts about fat.

FACT: Fat-free does not equal calorie-free. Many non-fat or low-fat foods have very high levels of sugar, which often significantly increases the calorie content of foods. In addition, people tend to eat larger portions of fat-free foods, thereby increasing the amount of calories consumed.

FACT: Fat satiates. In general, you need to eat less of a food with fat than you do of a non-fat food to feel full. For this reason, many people tend to overeat non-fat or low-fat foods.

FACT: You *need* some fat. This one is hard for people to accept, but it is true. Fat is a major nutrient that is vital for proper growth and development and maintenance of good health. Certain vitamins (A, E, and K) are soluble only in fat.

However, not all fats are healthful. In general, you should steer clear of saturated fats, which are artery cloggers. You'll find them in butter, meats, and palm and coconut oils. You should also avoid trans-fatty acids (fats that are formed when foods are hydrogenated and that are found in deep-fried commercial foods and many packaged foods, especially baked goods). These fats act like saturated fats but are even worse: In addition to raising levels of so-called "bad" cholesterol (known as LDL) in our bodies (as saturated fats do), they lower the levels of the "good" cholesterol (HDL) necessary to keep our arteries clear.

Monosaturated and polyunsaturated fats are the "good" fats. They're found in foods including olive oil and canola oil and are absolutely necessary for many functions of life. Our bodies also require essential fatty acids (EFAs), such as linoleic and alpha linoleic acid, for normal cell growth and development. The only way to get these fatty acids is through your diet. EFAs are found primarily in fatty fish, such as salmon and mackerel, and in certain nuts, oils, and dark green vegetables. There is significant evidence that a diet rich in essential fatty acids can protect against heart disease. Recently, the American Heart Association, in recognition of the important heart protective role that these fatty acids play, revised its dietary guidelines to include suggesting that we eat two servings of fatty fish each week.

Recommended daily intake of fat is 30 to 65 grams per day (approximately 25 to 30 percent of your total caloric intake).

THE FOOD GUIDE PYRAMID

The Food Guide Pyramid provides a visual depiction of the types and quantities of foods you should eat every day. It is broken into six food groups: grains, vegetables, fruits, dairy, proteins, and fats, oils, and sweets. Most of your diet should come from the foods at the base of the Pyramid (the grains group); the least amount should come from those at the top (fats, oils and sweets). You'll notice that you can have six to 11 servings of grains each day, which are rich in carbohydrates.

What Counts as a Serving?

The Food Guide Pyramid tells us to eat a particular number of servings per day of each kind of food: 3 servings of meat, 3 servings of milk, and so forth. But what exactly is one serving?

Milk, Yogurt, and Cheese

Eat 2 to 3 servings every day

1 serving equals 1 1/2 ounces of natural cheese OR 2 ounces of process cheese OR 8 ounces of yogurt OR 8 ounces of milk.

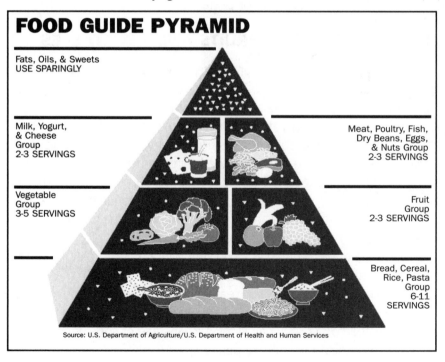

FOOD GUIDE PYRAMID

Fats, Oils, & Sweets
USE SPARINGLY

Milk, Yogurt,
& Cheese
Group
2-3 SERVINGS

Meat, Poultry, Fish,
Dry Beans, Eggs,
& Nuts Group
2-3 SERVINGS

Vegetable
Group
3-5 SERVINGS

Fruit
Group
2-3 SERVINGS

Bread, Cereal,
Rice, Pasta
Group
6-11
SERVINGS

Source: U.S. Department of Agriculture/U.S. Department of Health and Human Services

197

Meat, Poultry, Fish

Eat 2 to 3 servings every day

1 serving equals 2 to 3 ounces of cooked lean meat, poultry, or fish. 1/2 cup of cooked dry beans OR 1 egg OR 2 tablespoons peanut butter count as 1 *ounce* of lean meat.

Vegetables

Eat 3 to 5 servings every day

1 serving equals 1 cup of raw leafy vegetables OR 1/2 cup of other vegetables, cooked or chopped raw OR 3/4 cup of vegetable juice.

Fruit

Eat 2 to 4 servings every day

1 serving equals 1 medium apple, banana, or orange OR 1/2 cup of chopped, cooked, or canned fruit OR 3/4 cup of fruit juice.

Cereal, Rice, and Pasta

Eat 6 to 11 servings every day

1 serving equals 1 slice of bread OR 1 ounce of ready-to-eat cereal OR 1/2 cup of cooked cereal, rice, or pasta.

THE IMPORTANCE OF FRUITS AND VEGETABLES

In addition to choosing healthy grains, try to eat at least five servings of fruits and vegetables every day. This is essential. Many scientific studies have shown that people whose diets are plentiful in fruits and vegetables have reduced risk for many diseases, including a variety of cancers. Fruits and vegetables are great sources of essential vitamins, minerals, and fiber. Unfortunately, most of us do not eat the five recommended servings daily; and if we do, we eat the less healthy vegetables, such as iceberg lettuce, rather than the nutrient-dense dark greens. Dark green leafy vegetables, deeply colored fruits, and beans and peas are very rich in vitamins and minerals. A good rule of thumb is to make your plate as colorful as possible with a variety of vegetables to be sure you are getting all the nutrients you need.

How can you make sure you eat enough from this food group? Choose chopped vegetables as a snack when you feel hungry; or grab an apple instead of a candy bar. Drink juice instead of soda. Prepare salads with tomatoes, cucumbers, peppers, and other vegetables. Soon you'll see how easy it really is to eat those five servings.

WATER

Water, which comprises about 75 percent of our total body weight, serves many functions. It helps regulate our body temperature. When we sweat, we rid ourselves of excess heat. Water transports needed nutrients to our cells and removes toxic substances and wastes. It cushions our body tissues and lubricates our joints. Water provides moisture for our respiratory system and is essential for our digestion. Since water is a major component of all cell structures, including muscle structure and function, it takes second place only to oxygen as the most important body component. Unfortunately, most people often overlook this fact.

Since we cannot store or conserve water, it is critical to drink adequate amounts of it every day, especially in hot weather and during physical training. In general, you should consume up to four quarts a day (that's 12 to 16 8-ounce glasses). Ideally you should drink water in intervals throughout the day. Keep a bottle with you at all times. Keep it at your desk so that you can easily take regular drinks. When you exercise you should drink one to two cups of water an hour before you begin and then an additional four to eight ounces every 15 minutes during your workout.

Substances such as alcohol, caffeine, and tobacco increase your body's need for water. Consumed in excess, these substances will harm your body and hinder your performance. Not drinking enough water during physical training or on hot days can result in lack of coordination, irritability, fatigue, muscle cramping, mental confusion—and even more severe problems. Water intake is vital, so stay hydrated!

VITAMINS AND MINERALS

When it comes to supplementing our diets with vitamins people can be passionate. Some people strongly believe that taking a large number of vitamins each day is necessary to maintain or improve their health. However, vitamins are not subject to Food and Drug Administration (FDA) approval, and so manufacturers have wide leeway in marketing these products. You should be careful about taking any vitamins in very large doses (100 times the RDA) as they can be toxic at these levels.

Vitamins and minerals are found in the foods we eat and most nutrition experts agree that the best way to get vitamins is by eating a healthy diet. So, if you eat a healthy diet based on the Pyramid guidelines you probably will get all the vitamins and minerals you need.

However, many of us because of poor eating habits, have developed deficiencies—most often in folate, vitamin B6, antioxidants, calcium, and zinc. Taking a daily multivitamin—one that does not exceed the recommended nutrient levels—may be a good way to insure that you are receiving adequate amounts of these nutrients.

Antioxidants are important compounds that preserve and protect your body's cells from the damage of free radicals. Free radicals are oxygen molecules that have split into single electron molecules and can cause tissue damage. Beta carotene, vitamins C and E, and the minerals sulfur and selenium are powerful antioxidants. The following chart provides the US Recommended Daily Allowance for the major vitamins and minerals for adults. Bear in mind that your age and certain health conditions may call for you to have more or less of a particular vitamin or mineral. Check with your doctor.

VITAMINS

VITAMIN A
FUNCTIONS
Prevents night blindness, keeps body tissues healthy, allows for normal bone and teeth growth

BEST FOOD SOURCES
Dark, green leafy vegetables, red, orange, or yellow vegetables and fruits, liver, eggs, fish oils, and fortified foods such as milk

REQUIREMENTS
800 to 1000 micrograms retinol equivalents

DEFICIENCY
Poor night vision, increased risk of osteomalacia (soft bones), and osteoporosis

TOXICITY
Liver damage, bone abnormalities, headaches, double vision, hair loss, vomiting

VITAMIN D
FUNCTIONS
Promotes strong bones and teeth

BEST FOOD SOURCES
Eggs, cheese, sardines, fortified milk, cereals

REQUIREMENTS
5 to 10 micrograms

DEFICIENCY

Increased risk of osteoporosis and osteomalacia

TOXICITY

Weak muscles and bones, kidney stones, excessive bleeding

VITAMIN E

FUNCTIONS

Helps form cell membranes, increases resistance to disease and possibly reduces the risk of certain cancers as well as heart disease

BEST FOOD SOURCES

Vegetable oils, seeds, nuts, and wheat germ

REQUIREMENTS

8 to 10 mg alpha-tocopherol equivalents

DEFICIENCY

Abnormal nervous system functioning, premature very low birth weight infants

TOXICITY

Unknown but very high amounts may interfere with the functioning of other nutrients

---

VITAMIN K

FUNCTIONS

Promotes normal blood clotting

BEST FOOD SOURCES

Green leafy vegetables

REQUIREMENTS

55 to 80 micrograms

DEFICIENCY

Abnormal blood clotting

TOXICITY

None known

VITAMIN C

FUNCTIONS

Repairs damaged tissues, promotes wound healing, increases resistance to infection, maintains healthy gums, bones, and teeth

BEST FOOD SOURCES

Citrus fruits and juices, tomatoes, potatoes, and raw cabbage

REQUIREMENTS
60 milligrams

DEFICIENCY
Scurvy (symptoms may include bleeding, improper wound healing, loose teeth, and swollen gums)

TOXICITY
Gastrointestinal pain and diarrhea

VITAMIN B1 (THIAMIN)

FUNCTIONS
Carbohydrate metabolism

BEST FOOD SOURCES
Whole grains, nuts, peas, beans, pork, enriched breads and cereals

REQUIREMENTS
1 to 1.5 micrograms

DEFICIENCY
Weak muscles, nerve damage, fatigue

TOXICITY
None known

VITAMIN B2 (RIBOFLAVIN)

FUNCTIONS
Energy release and cell repair

BEST FOOD SOURCES
Poultry, enriched breads, cereals and grains, as well as green leafy vegetables, organ meats, cheese, milk, and eggs

REQUIREMENTS
1.2 to 1.8 milligrams

DEFICIENCY
Sore red tongue, dry flaky skin, cataracts

TOXICITY
None known

NIACIN (NICOTINIC ACID)

FUNCTIONS
Allows cells to use fuel and oxygen

BEST FOOD SOURCES
Meat, fish, poultry, nuts, legumes, enriched cereals and whole grains

REQUIREMENTS

13 to 20 milligrams

DEFICIENCY

Pellagra (symptoms may include dermatitis, diarrhea, and dementia)

TOXICITY

In very high doses, flushed skin, possible liver damage, high blood sugar, and stomach ulcers

---

VITAMIN B6 (PYRIDOXINE)

FUNCTIONS

Assists in protein and red blood cell formation, helps produce antibodies and hormones

BEST FOOD SOURCES

Meat, chicken, fish, nuts, legumes, and whole grains

REQUIREMENTS

1.5 to 2 milligrams

DEFICIENCY

Dermatitis, anemia, convulsions, and nausea

TOXICITY

nerve damage

FOLATE (FOLACIN OR FOLIC ACID)

FUNCTIONS

Produces DNA and RNA to make cells, helps make red blood cells

BEST FOOD SOURCES

Dark green leafy vegetables, orange juice, dried beans, liver, whole grain breads, and cereals

REQUIREMENTS

180 to 200 micrograms

DEFICIENCY

Increased risk of spina bifida in offspring, weakness, irritability, sore red tongue, diarrhea, weight loss, anemia

TOXICITY

Can mask B12 deficiency, which if untreated, can cause permanent nerve damage

VITAMIN B12 (COBALAMIN)
FUNCTIONS
Assists in DNA, RNA and nerve formation, helps make red blood cells, facilitates energy metabolism
BEST FOOD SOURCES
Meat, poultry, fish, dairy products, and fortified foods
REQUIREMENTS
2 micrograms
DEFICIENCY
Numb hands and feet, fatigue, anemia
TOXICITY
none known

BIOTIN
FUNCTIONS
Assists in energy production
BEST FOOD SOURCES
Eggs, liver, dried beans, nuts, whole grains and cereals
REQUIREMENTS
30 to 100 micrograms
DEFICIENCY
Loss of appetite, fatigue, dry skin, heart abnormalities and depression
TOXICITY
None known

PANTOTHENIC ACID
FUNCTIONS
Assists in energy production
BEST FOOD SOURCES
Meat, poultry, fish, whole grains, and legumes
REQUIREMENTS
4 to 7 milligrams
DEFICIENCY
Numb hands and feet
TOXICITY
Diarrhea and water retention

MINERALS

CALCIUM
FUNCTIONS
Required for blood clotting, nerve, muscle, and cell membrane functions, builds bone and teeth, promotes enzyme reactions
BEST FOOD SOURCES
dairy products, green leafy vegetables, tofu, almonds, and legumes
REQUIREMENTS
800 to 1200 milligrams
DEFICIENCY
Increased risk for osteoporosis
TOXICITY
Kidney stones and damage, constipation

PHOSPHORUS
FUNCTIONS
Promotes bone, teeth, DNA, and RNA growth, assists in energy production
BEST FOOD SOURCES
Meat, poultry, fish, eggs, legumes, nuts, and breads
REQUIREMENTS
800 to 1200 milligrams
DEFICIENCY
Bone loss, weakness, loss of appetite and pain
TOXICITY
Decreases calcium levels in the blood leading to bone loss

MAGNESIUM
FUNCTIONS
Component of bones and many enzymes, needed for energy production, muscle contractions, normal nerve and muscle cell functioning
BEST FOOD SOURCES
Whole grains, legumes, nuts
REQUIREMENTS
280 to 400 milligrams
DEFICIENCY
Muscle tremors, poor coordination, nausea, weakness, convulsions, and poor appetite

TOXICITY
Nausea, low blood pressure, heart abnormalities, vomiting

CHROMIUM
FUNCTIONS
Allows body to use glucose
BEST FOOD SOURCES
Nuts, whole grains, and meat
REQUIREMENTS
50 to 200 micrograms
DEFICIENCY
Nerve damage and high blood sugar
TOXICITY
None known

COPPER
FUNCTIONS
Facilitates energy production, component of enzymes, helps form hemoglobin and connective tissue
BEST FOOD SOURCES
Fruits, vegetables, nuts, seeds, legumes, liver
REQUIREMENTS
1.5 to 3 milligrams
DEFICIENCY
Anemia
TOXICITY
Liver damage, coma, nausea, vomiting, and diarrhea

FLOURIDE
FUNCTIONS
Prevents tooth decay, strengthens bones
BEST FOOD SOURCES
Sardines, salmon, fluoridated water, and tea
REQUIREMENTS
1.5 to 4 milligrams
DEFICIENCY
Tooth decay
TOXICITY
Brittle bones, stained or mottled teeth

IODINE
FUNCTIONS
Forms hormones that regulate the rate of energy usage
BEST FOOD SOURCES
Seafood and table salt
REQUIREMENTS
150 micrograms
DEFICIENCY
Enlarged thyroid and weight gain
TOXICITY
Enlarged thyroid

IRON
FUNCTIONS
Component of hemoglobin that carries oxygen to the cells
BEST FOOD SOURCES
Meat, poultry, fish, legumes, green leafy vegetables, dried fruits, and legumes
REQUIREMENTS
10 to 15 milligrams
DEFICIENCY
Infections, anemia, and fatigue
TOXICITY
Poisonous to children; may lead to hemochromatosis

MANGANESE
FUNCTIONS
A component of enzymes involved in energy and protein metabolism
BEST FOOD SOURCES
Whole grain products, tea, fruits, and vegetables
REQUIREMENTS
2 to 5 milligrams
DEFICIENCY
Rare
TOXICITY
Nerve damage

MOLYBDENUM
FUNCTIONS
Component of enzymes
BEST FOOD SOURCES
Organ meats, milk, legumes, and whole grains
REQUIREMENTS
75 to 250 micrograms
DEFICIENCY
Rare
TOXICITY
May interfere with copper use

SELENIUM
FUNCTIONS
Protects cells from damage, assists with cell growth
BEST FOOD SOURCES
Seafood, meats, grains, and seeds
REQUIREMENTS
50 to 70 micrograms
DEFICIENCY
May damage the heart
TOXICITY
Nerve damage, fatigue, irritability, nausea, vomiting, diarrhea, stomach pain

ZINC
FUNCTIONS
Needed for wound healing, growth, reproduction, carbohydrate, protein, and alcohol metabolism, and the making of DNA and RNA
BEST FOOD SOURCES
Meat, liver, eggs, dairy, whole grains, legumes, and oysters
REQUIREMENTS
12 to 15 milligrams
DEFICIENCY
Loss of senses of taste and smell, loss of appetite, reduced resistance to infection, scaly skin, growth retardation
TOXICITY
Interferes with copper absorption and immune functioning, reduces good blood cholesterol (HDL), upsets stomach, and may cause nausea and vomiting

SODIUM

FUNCTIONS
Regulates fluids, blood pressure, nerve and muscle function

BEST FOOD SOURCES
Processed foods and table salt

REQUIREMENTS
Minimum of 500 milligrams

DEFICIENCY
Muscle cramps, dizziness, nausea, and fatigue

TOXICITY
May cause high blood pressure

POTASSIUM

FUNCTIONS
Fluid and mineral balance, blood pressure regulation, nerve and muscle function

BEST FOOD SOURCES
Fruits, vegetables, poultry, meat, and fish

REQUIREMENTS
Minimum of 2000 milligrams

DEFICIENCY
Abnormal heartbeat, muscle paralysis, weakness, lethargy

TOXICITY
Heart abnormalities

CHLORIDE

FUNCTIONS
Component of stomach acid, regulates fluid balance

BEST FOOD SOURCES
Table salt

REQUIREMENTS
Minimum of 750 milligrams

DEFICIENCY
Growth failure, behavioral and learning problems, poor appetite

TOXICITY
May cause high blood pressure

READING FOOD LABELS

Nutrition Facts

Serving Size 1 oz. (2 cups 28g)
Servings Per Container about 1

Amount Per Serving

Calories 130	Calories from Fat 60	
		% Daily Value*
Total Fat 6g		**10%**
Saturated Fat 1g		**5%**
Polyunsaturated Fat 1g		
Monounsaturated Fat 1g		
Cholesterol 0mg		**0%**
Sodium 150mg		**5%**
Total Carbohydrate 17g		**6%**
Dietary Fiber 2g		**8%**
Sugars 1g		
Protein 2g		
Vitamin A		0%
Vitamin C		0%
Calcium		0%
Iron		10%

* Percent Daily Values are based on a 2,000 calorie diet. Your Daily Values may be higher or lower depending on your calorie needs:

		Calories:	2,000	2,500
Total Fat	Less than		65g	80g
Sat Fat	Less than		20g	25g
Cholesterol	Less than		300mg	300mg
Sodium	Less than		2,400mg	2,400mg
Total Carbohydrate		300g	375g	
Dietary Fiber			25g	30g

Ingredients: Corn Meal, Canola Oil, Aged Cheddar Cheese, (Milk, Salt, Cheese Cultures, Enzymes), Whey, Buttermilk, Maltodextrin, and Salt.

Learning how to interpret the information on food labels gives you a valuable nutrition tool. The ingredients listed first are the ones present in the highest concentrations by weight. Too often those ingredients are sugar and sodium. Shop for foods that have healthy ingredients front and center.

The serving sizes listed on labels can also be misleading, so you need to examine them carefully. For instance, the label on a small bag of potato chips may list "150 calories per serving," which doesn't sound like much. But read the label more carefully, and you may find that the bag contains *three* servings, not just one. If you eat all of the chips in the bag, you'll have consumed 450 calories.

Finally, it is helpful to know how to convert the nutrients presented on the label in grams to calories to determine how much (energy-wise) of each individual nutrient you would be eating in a serving.

Carbohydrates: 1 gram equals 4 calories
Proteins: 1 gram equals 4 calories
Fats: 1 gram equals 9 calories

When reading labels pay particular attention to the amount of cholesterol and sodium listed. You might be surprised by how many low-fat and low-calorie foods contain high levels of sodium (healthy adults should aim for a total intake of no more than 2,400 milligrams per day.) And check to see whether the food contains saturated or hydrogenated oils; if it does, you may want to avoid it because hydrogenated foods contain the unhealthy and potentially harmful trans-fatty acids.

RECRUITING INFORMATION

For more information about how to join the Pararescue or Combat Control teams, contact your local Air Force recruiter or write:

Pararescue/ Combat Control Selection Team
1780 Carswell Avenue, Suite 2
Lackland Air Force Base, Texas 78236-5506

or call:
Toll-free 1-800-438-2696

ABOUT THE AUTHORS

ANDREW FLACH

A lifelong fitness enthusiast, Andrew was born and raised in New York City, and is a graduate of St. David's School, The Browning School, and Vassar College. When he is not running a multi-million dollar media business, his recreational pursuits include sailing, mountaineering, rock climbing, mountain biking, SCUBA diving, and flying. He still resides in New York City.

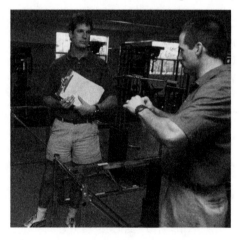

PETER FIELD PECK

Peter Field Peck is a freelance photographer. His work has appeared nationally in newspapers, magazines, and books. He currently resides in New York City.

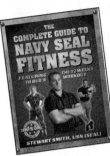
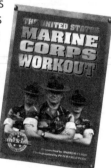

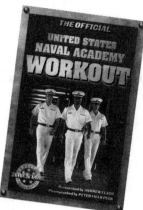

Have questions about this workout?

Ask the author at:

www.getfitnow.com

The hottest fitness spot on the Internet!

Home of:

Featuring

"Ask the Expert" Question and Answer

Boards

Stimulating Discussion Groups

Cool Links

Great Photos and Full Motion Videos

Downloads

The Five Star Fitness Team

Hot Product Reviews

And more!

Log on today to receive a FREE catalog or call us at

1-800-906-1234

The Official Five Star Fitness Series
A Getfitnow.com Book

Hatherleigh Press/Getfitnow.com Books
5-22 46th Avenue, Suite 200
Long Island City, NY 11101
1-800-528-2550
Visit our website: www.getfitnow.com

**Before beginning any strenuous exercise program consult your physician. The
author and publisher of this book and workout disclaim any liability, personal or
professional, resulting from the misapplication of any of the training procedures
described in this publication.**

All Getfitnow.com titles are available for bulk purchase, special
promotions, and premiums. For more information, please contact the manager
of our Special Sales Department at 1-800-528-2550.

Library of Congress Cataloging-in-Publication Data
Flach, Andrew, 1961–
The official United States Air Force elite workout / researched by Andrew Flach;
photographed by Peter Field Peck.
p.   cm. -- (Official Five Star fitness guides)
ISBN 978-1-57826–174–1 (alk. paper)
1. Exercise for men. 2. Physical fitness for men. 3. United States. Air Force.
I. Title. II. Series: Flach, Andrew, 1961–
Official Five Star fitness guides.
GV482.5.F53   1999
613.7'0449--dc21   99–28830
                                                    CIP

Cover design by Gary Szczecina
Text design and composition by DC Designs
Photographed by Peter Field Peck
with Canon® cameras and lenses on Kodak® and Fuji® print and slide film
Underwater images photographed with Nikonos IV

Printed on acid-free paper
10 9 8 7 6 5 4 3

THE OFFICIAL UNITED STATES AIR FORCE ELITE WORKOUT

RESEARCHED BY
ANDREW FLACH

PHOTOGRAPHED BY
PETER FIELD PECK

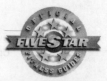

GETFITNOW.COM BOOKS
NEW YORK